THE
TRACKS
WE LEAVE

ETHICS IN HEALTHCARE
MANAGEMENT

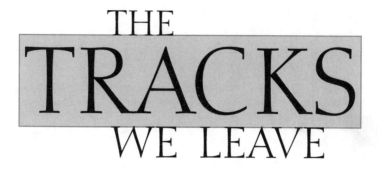

THE
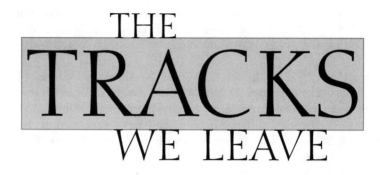
TRACKS
WE LEAVE

ETHICS IN HEALTHCARE
MANAGEMENT

FRANKIE PERRY

Health Administration Press

Library of Congress Cataloging-in-Publication Data

The tracks we leave : ethics in healthcare management / Frankie Perry.
    p.   cm.
    Includes bibliographical references and index.
    ISBN 1-56793-167-7 (alk. paper)
    1. Managed care plans (Medical care)—Moral and ethical aspects.
2. Medical ethics.   I. Perry, Frankie.
RA413.T73 2001
362.1'04258—dc21   2001039275

The paper used in this publication meets the minimum requirements of American National Standards for Information Sciences—Permanence of Paper for Printed Library Materials, ANSI Z39.48-1984. ∞™

Acquisitions Editor: Marcy McKay; Editor: Diana Flynn; Cover design: Betsy Perez

Health Administration Press
A division of the Foundation of the
  American College of Healthcare Executives
One North Franklin Street
Chicago, IL 60606
312/424-2800

We will be known forever by the tracks we leave.

Native American Proverb

CONTENTS

FOREWORD

FRANKIE PERRY has succeeded in creating an ethics book that is practical, pragmatic, and thought provoking. The judicious use of actual cases, issue discussions, and thoughtful brief essays on related topics makes for interesting and meaningful reading. This book not only serves the individual reader, but also provides the basis for roundtable and classroom discussions. An epilogue, rare in books of this type, provides some closure on each of the cases. This is real life tied together with solid contributions to our literature to help all of us improve our perspective on ethical situations.

This book is quite timely. Complications in healthcare delivery, complex business transactions, conflicts of interest, and the vastly expanding list of issues relating to bias confound our daily life as healthcare executives. Every organization faces these and other ethical problems constantly. Understanding these problems and acting proactively to prevent them is a critical skill of any executive. The breadth of this book goes far beyond the cases and provides a foundation for enhancing existing ethics education programs or creating new ones. Once read, this book will be a very useful reference tool for any institution's effort to deal with and prevent ethical dilemmas. Furthermore, this book should find a home in many graduate and undergraduate classes as both a text and a foundation for case discussions.

Creating a book of this type requires a special person. Frankie Perry approached this effort with outstanding preparation. Ms. Perry has held hospital positions from staff nurse through nursing supervision to top hospital management. From her hospital executive role, she joined the staff of the American College of Healthcare Executives (ACHE). Once again, she rose through the ranks to serve the professional society as executive vice president and as staff representative to the ACHE ethics committee. Implementing and preserving the ACHE *Code of Ethics* is the focus of the work of the ethics committee, which in turn becomes a major part of the role of the staff representative. This includes extensive analysis and action over violations of the *Code*. This is the exceptional perspective of Frankie Perry, which serves as a key to the value of this excellent book.

I have high hopes for this book and its effect on our profession, both in the practice and academic communities. I know it will assist all readers to more effectively fulfill their responsibilities as healthcare executives, as professionals in other healthcare roles, or as students aspiring to leadership and service roles in healthcare.

Stuart A. Wesbury, Jr., Ph.D., LFACHE
April 2001

ACKNOWLEDGMENTS

MUCH HAS been written in the past decade about ethics and how it applies to healthcare management and delivery, for which I am grateful.

My 28 years of hospital experience, first as a nurse and then as an administrator, and several years as staff to the American College of Healthcare Executives Ethics Committee made it clear to me that much *needed* to be written to help guide healthcare managers to successfully navigate the sometimes murky paths to ethical decisions.

Significant contributions to the literature have been made by John Griffith, Austin Ross, John Worthley, Laura Nash, and others whose valuable work has found its way into my efforts for this book. To them I owe a debt of gratitude.

I humbly submit this work to the collection of ethics literature in the field for healthcare managers, knowing that much has been written, but also knowing there can never be too much written on this important subject.

PREFACE

EVOLUTION IS a progression of interrelated phenomena. Society is continuously evolving and as an institution of society, healthcare is evolving as well. Thoughtful men and women have studied this evolution and helped to develop rules of conduct for each new paradigm. Our sense of morality changes as well, and the old rules of moral behavior do not always apply. On a fundamental level, people need and want guidance and standards to help them "do the right thing."

Nowhere is this evolution more evident than in the complex field of healthcare management. Healthcare as a microcosm of society reacts and responds to societal events. Continual advances in technology, changes in healthcare financing, increasing consumer needs and expectations, the proliferation of socioeconomically induced health problems, the ever expanding public scrutiny and litigation all contribute to the significant complexity of healthcare. As such, the decision-making process in healthcare management has become more complicated and it is especially difficult for healthcare executives to feel confident that they are making ethically responsible decisions.

Amid this turmoil of constant change, healthcare executives frequently find themselves in uncharted waters where the ethical "rules" may be unclear. "Real-life" ethical dilemmas are complex. Rarely is there a single ethical issue to resolve. More often, numerous intertwined issues with many stakeholders with diverse values interested in the outcome clamor for attention. Ambiguities abound; resolutions to ethical dilemmas do not come easily.

The cases presented here reflect the realities of healthcare management, the diversity of special interests, and the competing values and the moral conflicts that challenge the healthcare executive. Each case is followed by a description of the ethics issues inherent in the case which is then followed by a discussion of these interrelated issues. In some cases, a relevant essay completes the chapter.

The Paradise Hills Medical Center case in Chapter 1 focuses on medical errors, truth telling, and autonomy. It is followed by "Deciding Values," an essay by Joan McIver Gibson, Ph.D.

The Qual Plus HMO case (Chapter 2) appears to focus on conflict of interest issues but in reality is exploring the issue of conflicting moral demands when an individual is asked to do something the person believes to be unethical or observes one in authority behaving in unethical ways. Essays on "Ethical Issues in Managed Care" by Richard H. Rubin, M.D., and on "Evaluating Healthcare Ethics Committees" by Rebecca A. Dobbs, Ph.D., complete the chapter.

The Rolling Meadows Community Hospital case (Chapter 3) explores the issues surrounding mentorship, sexual harassment, and gender discrimination and offers a discussion that highlights some of the ambiguities of "wrong doing."

Chapter 4's University Hospital case highlights some of the pitfalls of impairment and how it can compromise patient safety and graduate medical education. An essay on other ethical issues in graduate medical education by Clinton H. Dowd, M.D. completes this chapter.

The Hillside County Medical Center case by Glenn A. Fosdick, FACHE in Chapter 5 focuses on the ethical implications of workforce reductions. Hospitals in financial stress sometimes use the euphemism, "right sizing," but to the employee being laid off and the ones left behind to pick up the slack, it can be a disaster. This case looks at the issues involved and the leadership required to make ethically sound decisions when a hospital is in financial crisis.

Chapter 6 provides legal perspectives on each of the preceding cases by attorney Walter P. Griffin, Esq. He also discusses the differences between "illegal and unethical" and "legal but unethical" behaviors. Chapter 7 discusses the ethics of managing people and the interpersonal conflicts that exist and the ethical dilemmas that may ensue within the healthcare delivery system.

The epilogue provides follow-up on each of these cases for those who wish to know if and how the ethical issues were resolved and what happened then.

These cases and the discussions emanating from them are intended to stimulate thoughtful analysis and reflection on the part of the reader to successfully navigate the quagmire of ambiguity that ethical dilemmas can present.

INTRODUCTION

A HEALTHCARE manager will be confronted with ethical dilemmas on a daily basis. Most of the time, unconsciously, the manager will make the right decisions and will "do the right thing." For the most part, those involved in healthcare are decent, moral individuals who are attracted to the healthcare field because they wish to contribute something of value to society. In spite of this, errors in judgment, detrimental decisions, and unintentional mistakes are made. More often than not, mistakes are the result of the barrage of decisions that must be made by managers who are pressed for time and strained by the demands of the job. Decisions are frequently made without the benefit of the thoughtful reflection and the consultation of others that may be required.

Theoretical constructs and ethical decision-making frameworks abound, but as the busy practitioner knows only too well, the realities of time and place sometimes supercede their proper usage. The healthcare manager is expected to know the answers, to make decisions quickly and authoritatively, and to lead the staff down a path of moral integrity.

This book is intended to provide some practical guidance for healthcare managers who are confronted with these challenges. What is a useful thought process that healthcare managers can employ to make this task easier? What steps can be taken to move staff in the direction of ethically sound decisions?

The process suggested here to arrive at such decisions is a relatively simple one—a series of questions that the healthcare manager can ask to

Figure 1: Issues Wheel

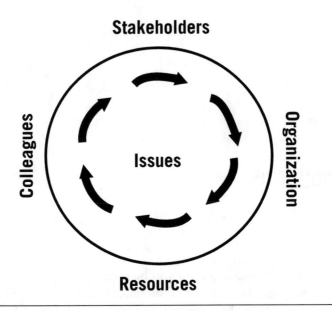

determine if additional time or resources need to be brought to bear on the decision-making process and the question at hand. These questions focus on identifying the issues, the stakeholders, the organizational impact, and the colleagues and resources available in any situation in question (see Figure 1).

- **Issues**
  What are the ethical issues in this situation? Relatively few single-issue situations exist. More often, a number of interrelated issues comprise the ethical dilemma. These must be isolated and *each* thoughtfully explored.

- **Stakeholders**
  What persons or groups will be affected by this situation and the actions taken? What will each feel is in his or her best interest?

- **Organization**
  What will be the effect on the organization that pays the executive's salary and has expectations that the executive will act in its best interests?

- **Colleagues**
  Which trusted colleagues can be consulted about this matter who may have insights, experiences, and knowledge to offer?—In confidence?

- **Resources**
  What resources are available? Does the organization have a mission statement? Values statement? Ethics committee? Ethics officer? Code of conduct? Compliance officer? Guiding principles? Policies? Laws? Regulations? Decision-making models? Legal counsel?

Caution must be exercised, however, to avoid the assumption that if no law or rule or regulation or policy addresses an action, then the action must be ethical. This is not true. Moral men and women do not need situations to "come with written instructions" to do the responsible thing.

Laura Nash in her article, "Ethics Without the Sermon" that appeared in *Harvard Business Review*, offers the following twelve questions for examining the ethics of a business decision:

1. Have you defined the problem accurately?
2. How would you define the problem if you stood on the other side of the fence?
3. How did the situation occur in the first place?
4. To whom and to what do you give your loyalty as a person and as a member of the corporation?
5. What is your intention in making this decision?
6. How does your intention compare with the probable results?
7. Whom could your decision or action injure?
8. Can you discuss the problem with affected parties before you make your decision?
9. Are you confident that your position will be as valid over a long period of time as it seems now?
10. Could you disclose without qualm your decision or action to your boss, your CEO, the board of directors, your family, society as a whole?
11. What is the symbolic potential of your action if understood? If misunderstood?
12. Under what conditions would you allow exceptions to your stand?[1]

John Worthley, citing L. T. Hosmer, discusses ten ethical principles that can be used to help healthcare executives determine an ethical course of action:

1. Self-interests: Never take any action that is not in the long-term self-interests of yourself and the healthcare organization to which you belong.

2. Personal virtues: Never take any action that is not honest, open, and truthful, and which you would not be proud to see reported widely in national newspapers and on television.

3. Religious injunctions: Never take any action that is not kind, and that does not build a sense of community.

4. Government requirements: Never take any action that violates the law.

5. Utilitarian benefits: Never take any action that does not result in greater good than harm in your healthcare facility.

6. Universal rules: Never take any action that you would be unwilling to see another healthcare professional take in similar situations.

7. Individual rights: Never take any action that abridges the agreed upon rights of others.

8. Economic efficiency: Always act to maximize profits subject to legal and market constraints and with full recognition of external costs.

9. Distributive justice: Never take any action in which the least among us are harmed in any way.

10. Contributing liberty: Never take any action that will interfere with the rights of others for self-fulfillment.[2]

Before codes of conduct and ethical frameworks for decision making were available, the young hospital administrators who reported to me looked for sage advice on how to do the right thing when they were on call. They knew if they really got into trouble, they could call me but that I expected them to have a plan of action when they did. To help them formulate this plan, I had given them four simple questions to apply to any situation:

1. What action is in the best interests of the patient(s) involved?

2. What action is in the best interests of the organization?

3. If this action is taken, what is the worst possible thing that can happen?

4. What is my contingency plan to deal with all possible ramifications of the action?

While every problem was not easily solved by using this thought process, my objective was to focus the administrator's thinking on what was best for the patient and the organization instead of subjective concerns like personal power, authority, or control in solving the problem at hand. For the most part, it worked, and the process did lend itself to the quick resolution of the kinds of problems that an administrator tends to see at three o'clock in the morning.

At the conclusion of Chapter 1, Joan McIver Gibson provides guidance in deciding values and applying values-based decision making to the analysis of ethics situations.

Regardless of which strategy the healthcare manager uses to arrive at a sound ethical decision, the manager must examine all of the consequences of each action considered.

The key to ethical decisions is an awareness on the part of the healthcare manager of the necessity of asking thoughtful questions and taking the time to formulate ethically sound answers. To do so will help healthcare managers to avoid hasty decisions that are not always attentive to the ethical implications of actions taken. Laura Nash reminds us that Aristotle said it well: "Contemplation is the best activity. It is also the most continuous since we can contemplate truth more continuously than we can perform any action."[3]

To further assist healthcare managers in future decision making, the Appendixes include:

American College of Healthcare Executives, *Code of Ethics*

American Hospital Association, Ethical Conduct for Healthcare Institutions

American College of Healthcare Executives Ethical Policy Statements for:

> Impaired Healthcare Executives
> Ethical Issues Related to Reduction in Force
> Ethical Decision Making for Healthcare Executives
> Creating an Ethical Environment for Employees

American College of Healthcare Executives Public Policy Statement for:

> Preventing and Addressing Harassment in the Workplace

Notes

1. Nash, L. 1981. "Ethics Without the Sermon." *Harvard Business Review* (November/December) 79–90.
2. Worthley, J. A. 1997. *The Ethics of the Ordinary in Healthcare*. Chicago: Health Administration Press. 234.
3. Nash, L. 1981. "Ethics Without the Sermon." *Harvard Business Review* (November/December) 83.

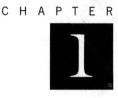

MEDICAL ERRORS:
PARADISE HILLS MEDICAL CENTER

P ARADISE HILLS Medical Center is a 500-bed teaching hospital in a major metropolitan area of the South. It is known throughout a tri-state area for its comprehensive oncology program and serves as a regional referral center for thousands of patients suffering from various forms of malignant disease.

Paradise Hills is affiliated with a major university and has residency programs in internal medicine, surgery, pediatrics, obstetrics/gynecology, psychiatry, radiology, and pathology, all fully accredited by the Accrediting Commission for Graduate Medical Education. In addition, Paradise Hills also has an oncology fellowship program, a university-affiliated nursing program, as well as training programs for radiology technicians and medical technologists. All of these teaching programs are highly regarded and attract students from across the nation.

Paradise Hills enjoys an enviable reputation throughout the area. It is known for its high-quality care, its state-of-the-art technology, and its competent, caring staff. While Paradise Hills is located within a highly competitive healthcare community, it boasts a strong market share for its service area. Indeed, its oncology program enjoys a 75 percent market share and its patients provide significant referrals to the surgery, pediatrics, and radiology programs as well.

Paradise Hills is a financially strong institution with equally strong leadership. Its past successes, in large part, can be attributed to its aggressive, visionary CEO and his exceptionally competent management staff.

But all is not as well as it seems to be at Paradise Hills. While the oncology program still enjoys a healthy market share, it has been slowly but steadily declining from its peak of 82 percent two years ago. In addition, the program's medical staff are aging and some of its highest admitting physicians are contemplating retirement. The oncology fellowship program was established a few years ago in anticipation of this, but unfortunately, thus far the graduates of this program have not elected to stay in the community. Of most concern to the CEO and his staff is the fact that the hospital's major competitor has recently recruited a highly credentialed oncology medical group practice from the Northeast and has committed enormous resources to strengthening its own struggling oncology program.

Last week the board of trustees for Paradise Hills had its monthly meeting with a fairly routine agenda. However, during review of a standard quality assurance report, one of the trustees asked for clarification of a portion of the report indicating that 22 oncology patients had received radiation therapy dosages in excess of what had been prescribed for them. The board was informed that the errors had occurred due to a flaw in the calibration of the equipment. The board was also informed that the medical physicist responsible for the errors had been asked to resign his position. The question was then asked if the patients who were recipients of the excessive radiation had been told of the error. The CEO responded that it was the responsibility of the medical staff to address this issue and it was their decision that the patients not be informed of the errors. The board did not concur that the responsibility for informing the patients of the errors rested solely with the medical staff and requested that the administrative staff review the hospital's ethical responsibility to these patients, as well as its liability related to this incident, and report back to the board within two weeks.

The CEO and his management staff responsible for the radiology department and the oncology program met with the medical staff department chairmen for internal medicine and radiology, the program medical directors for oncology and radiation therapy, and the attending oncologists. The CEO reported on the board discussion related to the incident and the board's request for a review of the actions taken, specifically the decision to not inform the affected patients.

The physicians as a whole agreed that the adverse effects of the accidental radiation overdose on the patients were unknown. Therefore, they argued the patients should not be told of the incident. These are cancer patients and they don't want or need any more bad news, the oncologists argued. "Let's face it, these patients are terminal." "Informing the patients of this error will only confuse them and destroy their faith and trust in their physicians and in the hospital," they added. Furthermore, they claimed, informing the patients of the errors may unnecessarily frighten them to the extent that they may refuse further treatment and that would be even more detrimental to them. Besides, argued the physicians, advising the patients of potential ill effects just might induce these symptoms through suggestion or excessive worry. Every procedure has its risks, insisted the chairman for radiology, and these patients signed an informed consent.

Physicians know what is best for their patients, the attending oncologists maintained, and they will monitor these patients for any ill effects. The department chairman for internal medicine volunteered that, in his opinion, this incident is clearly a patient-physician relationship responsibility and not the business of the hospital. Besides, added the chairman of radiology, informing the patients would "just be asking for malpractice litigation."

The medical director for the oncology program then suggested that the board of trustees and the management staff "think long and hard" about the public relations effect of this incident on the oncology program. "Do you really think patients will want to come to Paradise Hills if they think we're incompetent?", he asked.

The CEO conceded that he supported the position of the medical staff in this matter and he, too, was especially concerned about preserving the image of the oncology program, but "his hands were tied" since the board clearly considered this an ethical issue and one that would have to be referred to the hospital's ethics committee for its opinion.

The physicians noted that if indeed it was the subsequent recommendation of the ethics committee that these patients be informed, then realistically, that responsibility would rest with the patient's primary care physician and not with any of them.

ETHICS ISSUES

Truth Telling Is there a difference between lying to a patient and withholding the truth? Does it matter to the patient whether the act is one of omission or commission?

Justice and Fairness Is it fair to these patients to withhold information about their clinical treatment and any potential risks inherent in the accidental overdose?

A Patient's Right to Know Do these patients have a right to know about this incident? Can *not* informing the patients affected by this radiation overdose be reconciled with "A Patient's Bill of Rights"?

Adherence to the Hospital's Mission Statement, Ethical Standards, and Values Statement Are the actions considered related to this incident consistent with the hospital's mission statement, ethical standards, and values statement?

Adherence to Professional Codes of Ethical Conduct Are the actions considered related to this incident consistent with the codes of ethical conduct as promulgated by the professional organizations and associations representing physicians, healthcare executives, and hospitals?

Management's Role and Responsibility What is hospital management's role and responsibility in this matter? What is the role and responsibility specifically of the hospital CEO?

Legal Implications What are the legal implications of the actions being considered? To the hospital? To the physicians involved? Does the withholding of this medical treatment information and its potential risks from the patients involved constitute medical malpractice? In the view of the legal system, is this action indeed fraud? Has the hospital management considered the liability exposure for fraud which is not covered under medical malpractice insurance?

Other legal aspects to be considered relate to specific liability and issues of employment. Who employs and supervises the medical physicist? Who pays the medical physicist and who asked him to resign? Is the medical director for radiation oncology, who typically prescribes radiation therapy dosages, an employee of the hospital or an independent contractor? If the doctor is a contract physician does the contract stipulate that the medical physicist is hired and paid by the medical director? Should it? Is the medical director responsible for the actions of the medical physicist whether the medical physicist is employed by the medical director or not? Finally, who owns the Linear Accelerator used in this case?

Organizational Implications How will the actions being considered related to this incident impact the oncology program? The hospital as a whole? The hospital staff?

Ethical Decision-Making Frameworks Can the actions being considered related to this incident be justified within an acceptable ethical decision-making framework?

DISCUSSION

Truth Telling/Justice and Fairness

The fundamental issue in this case seems to be one of truth telling. Is it not a basic tenet of all ethical relationships that individuals and organizations tell the truth? Is it not the "right" thing to do?

The physicians in this case have argued that telling the truth would cause more harm than good; that not sharing this incident with their patients is, in fact, in their patients' best interest.

This, of course, assumes that the patients will never find out about the incident or that the patients will die without the incident ever coming to light. From a practical standpoint, this may indeed be the case. But upon closer examination, is this scenario likely or even probable? Sociologist John Denton reminds us that some 21 different hospital staff may interact with the patient in a single day.[1] In a teaching hospital, that number is likely to be compounded. The prescribed radiation therapy and the received radiation therapy are a matter of medical record. Incident reports and quality assurance reports are also a matter of record. Is it realistic to believe that staff will not have questions about the incident and, worst case scenario, inadvertently discuss it with an affected patient? Is it even possible with the great number of staff, physicians, and trustees who are privy to this information to maintain a "conspiracy of silence"? Is it right for the hospital to attempt to do this?

In the event that the patients or their families find out about the incident, after the fact, what then? What impact will this knowledge have on their opinions of the physicians and the hospital?

Clearly, human relationships depend on the communication of information. Without an honest sharing of information there can be no trust. Unfortunately, not telling the entire truth in a situation usually means additional shading of the truth or outright lying when questions arise. Typically, one lie begets another and yet another. Lying is, quite simply, self-destructive behavior, for once found out, liars are no longer trusted.[2]

In this case, lying or a withholding of the truth has enormous potential for undermining the image of the physicians and the hospital. If the knowledge of the incident is "discovered" by the patients or their families, the physicians and the hospital could be then accused of attempting to "cover-up" the incident. This could prove disastrous in the judgment of the community and in a court of law. Recent political scandals are a tragic reminder that the public will not stand for deceitfulness.

However, it could be argued that the intent here in withholding information is to protect the patients from unnecessary stress and anxiety, not unlike the "white lies" that one may use to spare someone's feelings in everyday life. Is this a fair comparison? Using the Golden Rule as a guide, if you or a loved one were the patient, would you want to know the truth about the incident? Or would you wish to be spared the anxiety?

In the assessment of Elizabeth Kubler-Ross, "the important question is not should I tell the truth, but how I should tell the truth, or how should I share information, important or not, with those who are asking me questions or who need to know what the truth is."[3] Does her assessment apply here?

Patient's Right To Know

Do the patients in this case have a right to know about the incident and how it may potentially effect them? A Patient's Bill of Rights as published by the American Hospital Association is publicly posted in Paradise Hills Medical Center. It states:

> Open and honest communication, respect for personal and professional values, and sensitivity to differences are integral to optimal patient care.
>
> Hospitals must ensure a healthcare ethic that respects the role of patients in decision making about treatment choices and other aspects of their care.
>
> The patient has the right to and is encouraged to obtain from physicians and other direct caregivers relevant, current, and understandable information concerning diagnosis, treatment and prognosis.
>
> Except in emergencies when the patient lacks decision making capacity and the need for treatment is urgent, the patient is entitled to the opportunity to discuss and request information related to the specific procedures and/or treatments, the risks involved, the possible length of recuperation, and the medically reasonable alternatives and their accompanying risks and benefits.[4]
>
> Bill of Rights, 2.

How do these standards of conduct apply to the radiation therapy incident at Paradise Hills? The management team and the physicians involved must review their applicability. In light of the fact that these standards are publicly posted, their review must take into consideration the patients' and their family members' interpretation of the standards, as well.

Do patients and their families have a right to know when a medical error has occurred during the course of their treatment? It seems the federal government is saying "yes."

Adherence to Hospital's Mission Statement, Ethical Standards, and Values Statement

In late 1999, the Institute of Medicine published a report entitled *To Err is Human: Building a Safer Health System* which claims that medical errors occurring in the nation's hospitals, clinics, and physician offices account for the deaths of nearly 100,000 Americans each year. As expected, this report was covered extensively by the media and this in turn prompted a rapid political response. Congressional hearings, a report from the Quality Interagency Coordination Task Force entitled *Doing What Counts for Patient Safety: Federal Actions to Reduce Medical Errors and Their Impact*, and a major policy speech on reducing medical errors by the president soon followed.

In his speech, President Clinton introduced a National Action Plan to reduce preventable medical errors by 50 percent within five years. This action plan called for:

- $20 million for the creation of a center for Quality Improvement in Patient Safety to sponsor research and education in reducing errors.
- New regulations requiring all 6000 hospital participants in the Medicare program to implement patient safety programs to reduce medical errors.
- Development of a national, state-based system for reporting medical errors that include mandatory reporting of preventable errors causing death or serious injury and voluntary reporting of other medical errors including "near misses."
- Support of legislation that protects provider and patient confidentiality without undermining existing tort remedies.
- New steps to specifically reduce medication errors.[5]

This National Action Plan signals governmental intervention in a domain that previously has been notorious for "policing its own" and where medical errors have been held in secret for fear of malpractice litigation and where those committing medical errors were blamed and punished and the prevailing standard for prevention of medical errors was to educate those involved in the hope that such errors would not happen again.

In an attempt to change what some have called a "conspiracy of silence," the Institute of Medicine and the Quality Interagency Coordinating Task Force recommended further actions including:

- Health plans involved in the Federal Employees Health Benefits Program must implement patient safety programs by 2001.
- Employers should incorporate patient safety performance into their healthcare purchasing decisions.
- Periodic relicensing and reexamination of physicians and nurses by state boards should include knowledge and competence in patient safety practices.
- Healthcare organizations should have a goal of continually improved patient safety.
- Proven medication safety practices should be implemented by healthcare organizations.
- Accrediting bodies such as the Joint Commission on Accreditation of Healthcare Organizations and others should review organizational efforts to minimize errors and promote patient safety.
- Computerized medical records should be implemented that are integrated with drug ordering and administrative systems.[6]

For healthcare providers, perhaps the most disconcerting of these recommendations is the mandatory reporting of medical errors to patients and their families. No responsible healthcare professional will argue with the need for strategies to reduce medical errors and provide assurances for patient safety. But the notion of placing the organization and its staff at risk for malpractice litigation gives one pause.

Yet, in the president's policy address he stated, "People should have access to information about a preventable medical error that causes serious injury or death of a family member, and providers should have protections to encourage reporting and prevent mistakes from happening again."[7] Is it reasonable to believe that this is possible, and more to the point, is the fear of litigation sufficient justification for withholding the truth from those affected by medical error?[8]

In fact, Kraman and Hamm argue that honesty may be the best policy in risk management. In their recent article in the *Annals of Internal Medicine*, they cite a study by Heckson and colleagues who found that of 127 families who sued their healthcare providers after perinatal injuries, 42 percent were motivated by suspicion of a cover-up or revenge.[9]

Kraman and Hamm reported on the experiences of one Veterans Affairs Medical Center that implemented a policy of full disclosure of medical errors to patients and families in the presence of a family attorney, if the family so desired. The medical center initiated this practice because staff believed it was the "right thing to do." They also found that this honest approach resulted in unanticipated financial benefits to the medical center when lower-cost settlements began replacing higher-cost litigation.[10]

Professional Codes of Ethical Conduct

Do the existing professional codes of ethical conduct promulgated by the professional organizations and associations representing physicians, healthcare executives, and hospitals require that the incident be fully disclosed to the patients?

Excerpts from the Code of Medical Ethics and Current Opinions of the Council on Ethical and Judicial Affairs published by the American Medical Association state:

> A physician shall deal honestly with patients and colleagues, and strive to expose those physicians deficient in character or competence, or who engage in fraud or deception.[11]
>
> The patient has the right to receive information from physicians and to discuss the benefits, risks, and costs of appropriate treatment alternatives. Patients should receive guidance from their physicians as to the optimal course of action. Patients are also entitled to obtain copies or summaries of their medical records, to have their questions answered, to be advised of potential conflicts of interests that their physicians might have, and to receive independent professional opinions.[12]

Excerpts from the American College of Healthcare Executives *Code of Ethics* state:

> The healthcare executive shall conduct all personal and professional activities with honesty, integrity, respect, fairness, and good faith in a manner that will reflect well on the profession.[13]
>
> The healthcare executive shall assure the existence of a process that will advise patients or others served of the rights, opportunities, responsibilities, and risks regarding available healthcare services.[14]

Excerpts from the American Hospital Association's Management Advisory on Ethics: Ethical Conduct for Health Care Institutions state:

> Healthcare institutions by virtue of their role as healthcare providers, employers, and community health resources have special responsibilities for ethical conduct and ethical practices that go beyond meeting minimum legal and regulatory standards. Their broad range of patient care, education, public health, social services, and business functions is essential to the health and well-being of their communities. These roles and functions demand that healthcare organizations conduct themselves in an ethical manner that emphasizes a basic community service orientation and justifies the public trust . . .[15]
>
> The governing board of the institution is responsible for establishing and periodically evaluating the ethical standards that guide institutional policies and practices. The governing board must also assure that its own policies, practices, and members comply with both legal and ethical standards of behavior. The chief executive officer is responsible for assuring that hospital medical staff, employees, and volunteers and auxilians understand and adhere to these standards and for promoting a hospital environment sensitive to differing values and conducive to ethical behavior.[16]

While the language in these ethical standards is somewhat general, the standards do provide guidance to those wrestling with this ethical dilemma. As professionals, each physician and executive must determine if his or her actions are consistent with their respective ethical standards.

The American Hospital Association's Advisory on Ethical Conduct for Health Care Institutions clearly delineates the ethical responsibilities of the governing board and the CEO lending credence to the argument that ethical matters involving patient-physician relationships are indeed the "business of the hospital."

Understanding the Medical Staff Perspective

It is not surprising, however, that the physicians involved in this case would feel otherwise. A basic understanding of the factors that contribute to the medical staff orientation helps to explain why physicians adamantly protect what they consider to be their professional province.

Typically, the physician enjoys the supreme position in the hospital organizational hierarchy. The physician generally establishes and maintains the rules that regulate most patient care in the hospital and it is only through the physician that the patient can access the healthcare system. Herbert Blumer suggests that all organizations "represent the application of somebody's definition of what the organization should be." It is the physician who sets the standards for patient care and who defines illness.[17]

The physician is granted the authority to define illness because the physician possesses "a body of knowledge that defines and constructs the roles to be played in the context of the institution."[18] Roles make it possible for institutions to exist. By virtue of the role the physician plays, he/she is inducted into specific areas of knowledge, not only in the narrower cognitive sense but also in the sense of norms, values, and even emotions. This knowledge may become so internalized that the physician considers the role "an inevitable fate for which (he/she) may disclaim responsibility." "I have no choice in the matter, I have to act this way because of my position."[19]

Physicians learn their roles through a complex socialization process that begins when they enter medical school. The rigors and expense of medical school, the admission requirements, the protégé system, and the collegial bonds of the medical profession all reflect occupational social-ization. Upon completion of medical school, the symbolic universe of the physician includes elaborate rights, obligations, standard practices, and a role-specific vocabulary. The physician is now socialized to play the role as definer of reality for the patient.[20]

The effects of this socialization on the moral reasoning of medical students is reflected in a study conducted by Herbert, Meslin, and Dunn at the University of Toronto and published in the *Journal of Medical Ethics* in 1992. Their research instrument presented four clinical vignettes and respondents were asked to list the ethical issues in each. The study assumes that physicians must recognize issues before they can behave appropriately. Students in all four medical school years participated in the research project. The first-year students completed the survey during their medical school orientation. The fourth-year students identified far fewer ethical issues than the first-year students. The researchers concluded that "these studies show(ed) a disturbing pattern; the ethical sensitivity of medical students seems to decrease with more time in medical school. Is this the consequences of medical socialization and is it harmful?" they asked.[21]

In any discussion of the role of the physician, some attention must be given to professionalism. Critical components of professionalism include autonomy and self-regulation. The source, structure, and characteris-tics of professionalism place professionals in a position of dominance. Professionalism is considered by many as the ultimate in occupational status and the physician is the prototype of professionalism.[22] There are some who will argue that the physician's position of dominance is justified. After all, they say, physicians must make life and death decisions. Advocates of patient self-determination claim that physician dominance is detrimental. But the greatest challenge to the physician's dominant role in healthcare has been managed care. At Paradise Hills, the physicians have not yet experienced the prevalence of managed care that exists in other parts of the country.

Given the occupational socialization and the professional dominance that the Paradise Hills physicians enjoy, it is not surprising that they tend to *believe* that matters of patient care fall strictly within their domain.

Hospital Management's Role and Responsibility

What is hospital management's role and responsibility in this case? What is the role and responsibility specifically of the hospital CEO? Strict adherence to a literal interpretation of the standards of ethical conduct promulgated by the American College of Healthcare Executives and the American Hospital Association as discussed earlier would indicate that the role of the CEO in this case is indeed burdensome and one in which the CEO must balance complex needs and conflicting interests. In the fulfillment of all the CEO's duties, the executive has responsibilities to the governing board, to the institution, to the medical staff, to the employees, to the community, to the patients, to the profession, and to self.

The CEO is mandated to carry out the policies of the governing board which includes ensuring compliance with the ethical standards approved by the board for the practices of the institution. The CEO, likewise, is charged with the responsibility for ensuring that the institution operates in ways that are consistent with its mission statement and its statement of values, assuming one exists. Indeed, Austin Ross in his book, *Cornerstones of Leadership for Health Services Executives* says that "The CEO's greatest source of support in preserving ethical conduct within the organization is the organizational mission."[23]

Partnering with the Medical Staff

Paradise Hills and its management staff have a strong working relationship with its medical staff. Its oncology physicians have been especially loyal and committed to Paradise Hills and in return, hospital management has provided the resources and technology needed for the physicians to practice state-of-the-art medicine. It has been a "win/win" situation for Paradise Hills. The CEO is now determined to arrive at a solution to this problem that will preserve the existing medical staff–management relationship. Not incidentally, he knows he must avoid alienating these community-based physicians whose patients are vital to the financial viability of the hospital.

It is generally accepted that leadership hospitals embrace the core belief that medical staff participation is essential to the successful operations and strategic planning of the institution. Management in such an institution enthusiastically integrates medical staff participation into its way of doing business, fosters ongoing dialog with physicians, and recognizes the medical staff as a needed resource. The CEO at Paradise Hills has worked to develop such an environment and is staunch in his resolve that the medical staff must be full and active participants in this ethical decision making. The CEO believes that a satisfactory solution to this incident must not violate confidentiality of patient information, must not infringe upon or threaten the patient-physician relationships, and must not precipitate a lawsuit. He knows that to secure these objectives he must work closely with the medical staff on this issue and avoid an adversarial confrontation. The physicians must be full partners in the analysis and resolution of the problem. Their voice in the proceedings must be heard and attended to. The outcome must be one in which they have been allowed to exercise some element of control.

Fortunately, the CEO at Paradise Hills is armed with the primary prerequisite to successful partnering with the medical staff: they trust him. Now, he knows that to successfully solve this ethical problem, he must be well prepared with solid facts, a well-thought-out rationale for actions, and a commitment and a plan to deal with all consequences of the actions taken.

The CEO and the management staff must also recognize that medical errors take their toll on the physicians and other staff that may be involved. In an organizational culture that emphasizes perfection, self-reproach, and accountability, guilt can affect a clinician's effectiveness in future patient care. Management must, therefore, take measures to assist staff in appropriately coping with medical errors.[24]

Leadership

In this case, as in all ethical matters, the CEO has enormous leadership responsibility. It is the CEO who is responsible for the ethical culture within the organization, implementing the standards of ethical conduct, and serving as an ethical role model for staff. While clinical professionals may bring their own codes of conduct to the workplace, it is management that must set the tone for how business is conducted, how professionals interact, and how patients are served.

Bennis and Namus are clear on this point. "The leader is responsible for the set of ethics or norms that govern the behavior of people in the organization. Leaders set the moral tone."[25]

William D. Hitt in his book, *Ethics and Leadership: Putting Theory Into Practice*, cites results of research studies that demonstrate that the ethical conduct of individuals in an organization is influenced greatly by their leaders. Hitt says that leaders have three basic obligations:

1. Achieve an understanding of ethics.
2. Serve as a role model in making ethical decisions.
3. Develop and implement a plan of action for promoting ethical conduct on the part of his or her staff.[26]

The significance of the leader as role model should not be underestimated. Schmidt and Posner conducted studies to identify the five primary factors that influence ethical conduct in organizations by rank. They were:

1. Behavior of superiors
2. Behavior of one's peers in the organization
3. Ethical practices of one's industry or profession
4. Society's moral climate
5. Existence of organizational policy[27]

Austin Ross in his book, *Cornerstones of Leadership for Health Services Executives,* states that "effective leadership is still the healthcare system's best hope for anchoring ethics, values, and social responsibility within organizations." He continues that "The CEO nurtures the organizational social conscience by being personally dedicated and committed to accomplishing an organizational mission based on good ethical conduct."[28] Ethical problems are a true managerial dilemma because they represent conflict between an organization's economic performance and its social obligations to parties both within and outside of the organization.[29] This case, like all ethical problems, requires that the CEO, his management team, and the medical staff think through the consequences of their actions on multiple dimensions using ethical analysis as well as economic and legal analysis.[30] While the task is complex and the conflicts may appear insurmountable, Bennis and Namus remind us that "Leaders are persons who are able to influence others; this influence helps to establish the organizational climate for ethical conduct; ethical conduct generates trust; and trust contributes substantially to the long-term success of the organization."[31]

Notes

1. Denton, J. A. 1978. *Medical Sociology.* Boston: Little, Brown and Co. 132.
2. Thiroux, J. P. 1986. *Ethics Theory and Practice.* New York: Macmillan Publishing Co. 165.
3. Kubler-Ross, E. 1969. *On Death and Dying.* New York: Macmillan Publishing Co. 262.
4. *A Patient's Bill of Rights.* 1992. Chicago: American Hospital Association.
5. William Clinton. 2000. "Remarks by the President on Medical Errors," [Online information retrieved 2/2/2000]. <http://www.ahrq.gov/wh22200rem.htm>

6. "Doing What Counts for Patient Safety: Federal Actions to Reduce Medical Errors and Their Impact." 2000. Report of the Quality Interagency Coordination Task Force.

7. William Clinton. 2000. "Remarks by the President on Medical Errors," [Online information retrieved 2/2/2000]. <http://www.ahrq.gov/wh22200rem.htm>

8. Ibid.

9. Kraman, S. S., and G. Hamm. 1999. "Risk Management: Extreme Honesty May Be the Best Policy." *Annals of Internal Medicine* 131 (12) 913–67.

10. Ibid.

11. *Principles of Medical Ethics.* 1994. Chicago: American Medical Association, Preamble, II.

12. *Fundamental Elements of the Patient/Physician Relationship.* 1993. Chicago: American Medical Association, I.

13. *Code of Ethics.* 1995. Chicago: American College of Healthcare Executives, Section I, B.

14. *Code of Ethics.* 1995. Chicago: American College of Healthcare Executives, Section II, A, 4.

15. *Ethical Conduct for Healthcare Institutions.* 1992. Chicago: American Hospital Association, Introduction.

16. Ibid.

17. Blumer, H. 1969. *Symbolic Interactionism, Perspective and Method.* Englewood Cliffs, NJ: Prentice-Hall. 58.

18. Berger, P. L., and T. Luckmann. 1967. *The Social Construction of Reality.* Garden City, NY: Anchor Books, Doubleday and Co. 67.

19. Berger and Luckmann, 76.

20. Berger and Luckmann, 91.

21. Herbert, P. C., E. M. Meslin, and E. V. Dunn. 1992. "Measuring the Ethical Sensitivity of Medical Students: A Study at the University of Toronto." *Journal of Medical Ethics* (18): 142–7.

22. Friedson, E. 1970. *Professional Dominance.* New York: Atherton Press, Inc. 185.

23. Ross, A. 1992. *Cornerstones of Leadership for Health Services Executives.* Ann Arbor, MI: Health Administration Press. 28.

24. Morreim, E. 2000. "Ethical Imperatives of Medical Errors." *Healthcare Executive* (July/August) 15(4): 56.

25. Bennis, W., and B. Namus. 1985. *Leaders: The Strategies for Taking Charge.* New York: Harper and Row. 186.

26. Hitt, W. D. 1990. *Ethics and Leadership: Putting Theory into Practice.* Columbus, OH: Battalle Press. 4.

27. Schmidt, W., and B. Posner. 1983. *Managerial Values in Perspective.* New York: American Management Association.

28. Ross, 30.

29. Hosmer, L. T. 1987. *The Ethics of Management.* Homewood, IL: Irwin, Inc.

30. Hosmer, 108.

31. Bennis and Namus, 186.

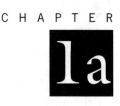

DECIDING VALUES

Joan McIver Gibson, Ph.D.

INTRODUCTION

Decisions whether to tell patients the "whole" story (including uncertainty, ambiguity, and "bad news"), honor professional responsibility, minimize legal liability, provide safe, quality care, and enhance programmatic and institutional financial health (not to mention survival) are values-based decisions. That is, they reflect what matters, in a given situation, to the decision maker(s).

Indeed, we would be hard pressed to come up with *any* decision or issue (public, private, or professional) that is not at bottom defined by *values*—that is, by our beliefs of what is useful, important, worthwhile, or desirable. Certainly this is the case with the issues at Paradise Hills Medical Center. So what should healthcare administrators, board members, and other managers, whose main "products" are decisions, do with this observation?

In a culture that still feels the effects of the nineteenth century positivist separation of "fact" from "value" we find ourselves without a robust language or strategy for seeing, naming, and working with

This chapter describes a values-based decision-making process and tool developed by Joan McIver Gibson and her colleague Mark Bennett, Decisions Resources, Inc. A book by these two authors, explaining the entire process and containing cases and work tools, is due to be published within the next year.

values. We are confident that as long as we are dealing with "facts" we can make progress. And so we search for "hard" data to lead the way. Would a right decision become clear if there were more conclusive data on the adverse effects of the accidental radiation, or if hospital policy were "black and white" regarding the ultimate decision makers on this issue, or if there were an in-depth analysis of projected market share over the next five years? Probably not. The decision maker(s) still must navigate a sea of conflicting interests and values.

As soon as someone raises the specter of a values discussion, however, many people fear a slide into the black hole of private, subjective, and interminable discussion. This is not helpful when things need to get done. This chapter introduces a process of values-based decision making for administrators and managers in healthcare institutions. It is, however, transferable to virtually every decision-making facet of our lives: professional, public, and private.

THEORY AND HISTORY

Are values really that separable from facts? Do values enter decision making only when we specifically invite them in? Scientists and philosophers over the past half century have dropped the fact/value dichotomy as at best outmoded and unhelpful, at worst—wrong. They observe that all reasoning, from the beginnings of language development through complex theory building, is the attempt to create, reflect on, and communicate *meaning*. Reasoning is the process of making meaning, or *valuing*. To label something as "factual" is already to make a very strong claim about its importance, status, utility, and reliability—that is, about its value.[1]

How do we go about discerning the values dimension of an issue or decision? What vocabulary do we need for capturing values and crafting decisions that *appropriately* reflect those values? Expanding our understanding of sources and types of values and their historical evolution in western philosophy may help.

VALUES: SOURCES AND TYPES

Professions, organizational culture, law, religion, social customs, family, and personal experience communicate important values (see Table 1a.1). What matters to us comes from the areas of strong influence in our lives. Consider the relative weight we place on these *sources* of interests and values. Sometimes, when faced with otherwise intractable conflicts among values, we make choices based on what we consider

Table 1a.1: Sources of Values

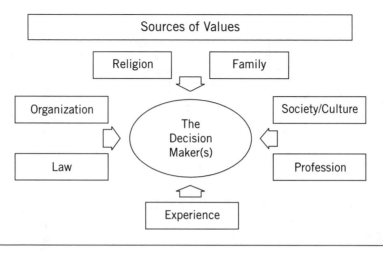

an influential source for values. For example, how should the Paradise Hills CEO weigh the relative influences of professional, personal, and community values? Should values issuing from one of these sources trump the others?

Another related strategy is to recognize that decision makers project various roles and approach decisions based on these roles. Cases present themselves differently, depending on the "disciplinary lens" through which we view them. Our roles grow out of our professional, social, and personal identities and entail specific perspectives or "lenses" that refract according to the *types* of values important to a given discipline or role. Consider the following perspectives:

- Legal: What does the law require?
- Scientific: Is the explanation comprehensive, coherent, and simple?
- Economic: Is this the best distribution of the resources available?
- Social: Does this policy respect the values and traditions of our diverse community?
- Aesthetic: Do things fit together and run efficiently and smoothly?
- Moral: Is it really the right thing to do?

This list is suggestive, not exhaustive, of ways to unpack, label, and reorganize the variety of interests and values embedded in a single issue or decision.

Table 1a.2: Examples of Values by Type

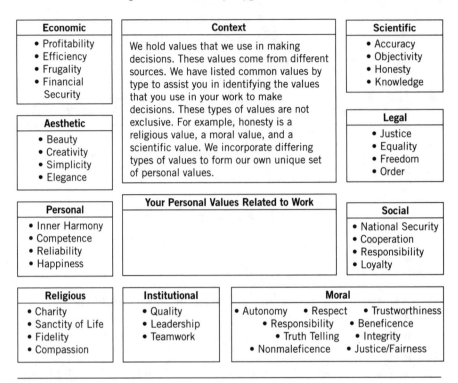

Economic	Context	Scientific
• Profitability • Efficiency • Frugality • Financial Security	We hold values that we use in making decisions. These values come from different sources. We have listed common values by type to assist you in identifying the values that you use in your work to make decisions. These types of values are not exclusive. For example, honesty is a religious value, a moral value, and a scientific value. We incorporate differing types of values to form our own unique set of personal values.	• Accuracy • Objectivity • Honesty • Knowledge

Aesthetic
• Beauty • Creativity • Simplicity • Elegance

Legal
• Justice • Equality • Freedom • Order

Personal	Your Personal Values Related to Work	Social
• Inner Harmony • Competence • Reliability • Happiness		• National Security • Cooperation • Responsibility • Loyalty

Religious	Institutional	Moral		
• Charity • Sanctity of Life • Fidelity • Compassion	• Quality • Leadership • Teamwork	• Autonomy • Responsibility • Truth Telling • Nonmaleficence	• Respect • Beneficence • Integrity • Justice/Fairness	• Trustworthiness

History of Values

Finally, *history* helps. In the United States, our contemporary set of values is a microcosm of 2000+ years of history. For example, reviewing our cumulative western (primarily Anglo-Saxon and European) heritage, we see certain markers along the way that signal different approaches to values. Understand that this tradition is but one of many cultural and historical strands that contribute to our American tapestry of values (see Table 1a.2).

In ancient Greece, at least for Plato and Aristotle, *virtue* mattered most (cf. today's "character counts" initiative). The question was: How do I personally cultivate virtuous character traits, that is, who should I *be*? rather than, what should I *do*? Plato and Aristotle believed that a morally good person with right desires, motivations, or intentions, is more likely to understand what should be done, more motivated to perform required acts, and more likely to form and act on moral ideals than someone without such virtuous traits.

At the beginning of the Christian era, two fundamental values were added: the *sanctity of life* and the importance of the *individual person*. Regardless of faith, the obligation to avoid harm and protect life, as well as the intrinsic worth of persons as autonomous agents are values and imperatives that continue to drive American law and social policy.

During the Renaissance and Enlightenment, *science, reason, and moral philosophy* joined forces. The scientific values of simplicity, coherence, and comprehensiveness in explanation were extended to other disciplines (e.g., social theory, religion, art). There was a deep faith in the power of reason and the promise of progress, and morality was an important—perhaps the primary—object of rational inquiry. Faith in reason as the guide to right action continues, even (perhaps especially) as we lament its absence.

In the twentieth century, the application of reason to moral values became more and more systematized, even as it was separated from scientific and "factual" inquiry. Just as science, in one of its dimensions, is systematized explaining, so moral philosophy (ethics) is systematized valuing. One way of doing this is by extracting and abstracting from individual cases, those evermore general and encompassing reasons, standards, and justifications for what constitutes right actions. These most general and broadly applicable standards we call *principles*. In medical ethics especially this system of analysis and decision making took hold.

A *principlist approach* to valuing and ethics:

- identifies the fundamental standards of right conduct, such as autonomy, respect for persons, beneficence, justice, truth telling, professional responsibility/integrity;
- argues the moral importance of such standards; and
- applies each (where necessary) to a given situation.

How we justify these principles and the actions they support is important. Do we look to these standards themselves for self-evident value, rather than to their consequences? Is there something about respect for persons and telling the truth that is intrinsically valuable, regardless of the circumstances or outcomes?

Should we calculate the consequences and seek the greatest good for the greatest number of people? The former approach is a *formalist* approach, the latter *utilitarian*. They are not mutually exclusive and both are helpful.

The task, however, is not simply and mechanistically to follow or apply certain principles (e.g., a Code of Ethics) to a given case, as one might follow a recipe, but rather to see how these standards help us understand and develop the moral dimension of a decision.

Toward the end of the twentieth century, as principlist ethics was focused on formulating and impartially applying universally binding moral principles, contemporary philosophers began to observe that universal principles are inadequate for practical guidance; that abstract formulations and hypothetical cases that separate moral agents from the particularities and uniqueness of their individual lives and circumstances, and moral problems from social, historical, contextual realities, are often less than helpful (see Table 1a.3).

For example, it is important to tell the truth. Yet, sometimes it is not clear what the truth is, or what meanings different "messengers" might communicate, or the degree to which quality patient care and safety might be compromised if a program is shut down. Unique circumstances, players, and environment are moving targets to be reckoned with. Context matters.

VALUES-BASED DECISION MAKING: A CONTEXTUAL APPROACH

A *contextual* (not to be confused with relativistic) approach to values-based decision making accommodates general principles, uniqueness, and particular details by focusing on *roles, relationships, and process*. The following elliptical diagram (Table 1a.4) illustrates the approach.

Features of the decision-making ellipse include: the importance of *context*, the *frames* we and others bring to a situation, working with values by *naming, clarifying*, and *weighing* them, *deciding* based on these values, and *communicating* accurately and thoroughly the decision and the reasons behind it as well.

Context

Cases arise and decisions are made in specific contexts. Decision makers must "see" the full context, history, tradition, current conditions, institutional values, as well as specific people, roles, and relationships that are at work. They must promote values and argue for their relative weight. Any decision involving Paradise Hills Medical Center must consider its history and role in the community, the current business climate, the institution's role as a teaching hospital, as well as the various roles and relationships of the respective players (physicians, CEO, board members, community at large). Effective decision makers understand the influence of context and use it to their advantage.

Table 1a.3: Major Historical Developments in Ethics

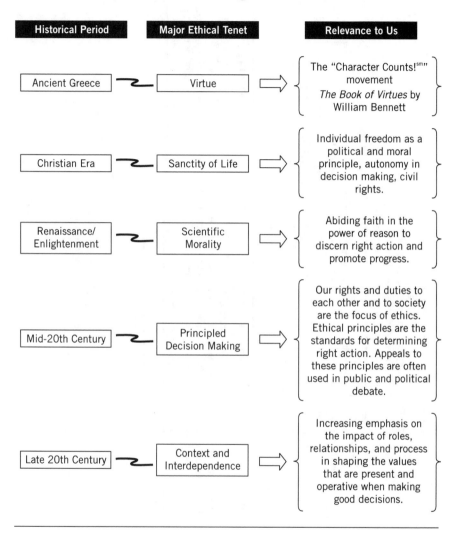

Historical Period	Major Ethical Tenet	Relevance to Us
Ancient Greece	Virtue	The "Character Counts!^{sm}" movement *The Book of Virtues* by William Bennett
Christian Era	Sanctity of Life	Individual freedom as a political and moral principle, autonomy in decision making, civil rights.
Renaissance/ Enlightenment	Scientific Morality	Abiding faith in the power of reason to discern right action and promote progress.
Mid-20th Century	Principled Decision Making	Our rights and duties to each other and to society are the focus of ethics. Ethical principles are the standards for determining right action. Appeals to these principles are often used in public and political debate.
Late 20th Century	Context and Interdependence	Increasing emphasis on the impact of roles, relationships, and process in shaping the values that are present and operative when making good decisions.

Framing: What Kind of Issue Do I Think This Is?

Each of us comes to any decision with a first "take" on what kind of issue it is. We might initially consider the Paradise Hills case to be an issue of public relations, or perhaps liability exposure, or program/institution survival, or professional fiduciary responsibility, or simply a matter of telling the truth. It is a virtual certainty that different parties will bring different initial frames to the decision. Frames are neither right or wrong,

Table 1a.4: "Decision-Making Ellipse"

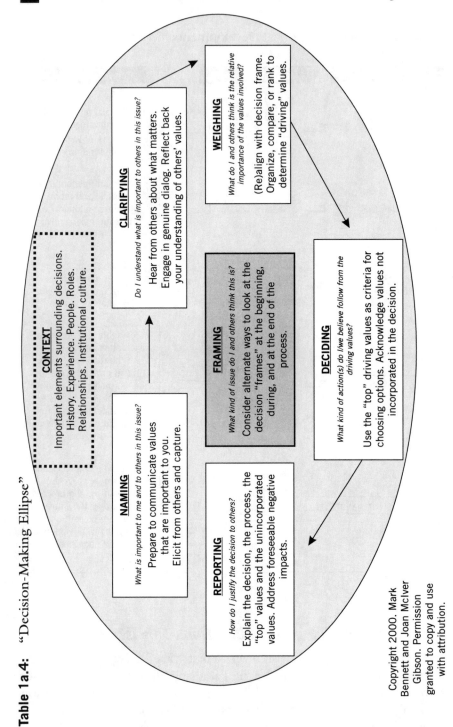

CONTEXT

Important elements surrounding decisions. History. Experience. People. Roles. Relationships. Institutional culture.

NAMING

What is important to me and to others in this issue?

Prepare to communicate values that are important to you. Elicit from others and capture.

CLARIFYING

Do I understand what is important to others in this issue?

Hear from others about what matters. Engage in genuine dialog. Reflect back your understanding of others' values.

WEIGHING

What do I and others think is the relative importance of the values involved?

(Re)align with decision frame. Organize, compare, or rank to determine "driving" values.

FRAMING

What kind of issue do I and others think this is?

Consider alternate ways to look at the decision "frames" at the beginning, during, and at the end of the process.

DECIDING

What kind of action(s) do I/we believe follow from the driving values?

Use the "top" driving values as criteria for choosing options. Acknowledge values not incorporated in the decision.

REPORTING

How do I justify the decision to others?

Explain the decision, the process, the "top" values and the unincorporated values. Address foreseeable negative impacts.

they simply "are." The Talmud reminds us that, "We see the world, not the way it is, but the way we are."

We need ways to simplify and structure all the information "noise" that surrounds us. Our brains are "hard-wired" to use categorical frames to bound what is "in" (relevant, important) and "out" (irrelevant, less important). Frames usually exist below our awareness and often remain untested and unexamined. They are not accessible for problem solving and decision making. Worse yet, they may impede our ability to see root causes of conflict. When frames are understood, appropriate, and flexible, they serve us well in dealing with difficult decisions and challenging situations. When they are hidden, unduly rigid, or based on flawed assumptions, they limit our ability to make wise decisions and may cause us to react to complex situations in an overly simplistic manner.

In decision making, frames determine who should participate, how the decision/question is formulated, what principles/values/standards are applicable, what information is relevant, what is at stake, what is the range of acceptable outcomes, and how we should treat each other.

The major task of the framing step is to consider alternative ways to define the problem or structure the question, both at the beginning and throughout the decision-making process. Key framing questions include: What kind of decision is this? What assumptions are we making? What boundaries do I/we/they put on this question? Who are the people involved?

Specific framing activities might include: Periodically stepping back during the decision process and asking if we have the question/issue/problem framed well; consulting with possible stakeholders about ways to frame the issue; listing three to five different ways to ask the question and getting feedback from key people about the best way to approach the problem.

Naming and Clarifying: Do I Understand What Is Important to Me and to Others in This Issue?

The real "brainstorming" part of this process involves identifying the interests and values held by stakeholders. The goal of this step is to generate a comprehensive list of values described in everyday language—always avoiding jargon. Questions that prompt useful "values answers" include: What really matters in this issue? What is important here that we really need to look at? What do you think our duties and obligations are in this situation? What worries you about this issue? When we look back on this decision one year from now, how will we know we did the right/best thing? If your teenager were watching us make this decision and asked why we did it, what would you say to her/him?

Answers to the question, "What is important?" might include: (1) that Paradise Hills Medical Center protect its good reputation; (2) that quality care and patient safety remain paramount; (3) that past, current, and future patients and families be able to trust the healthcare professionals at Paradise Hills; (4) that the hospital enjoy a strong economic position in the local healthcare community; and (5) that physicians honor their fiduciary duties to patients.

As values are named it is important for others to understand what they mean to the holder. Frequently our stated values are merely the visible tip of their larger meaning. Listening well, not merely waiting to speak, is essential. Skills for avoiding "serial monologues" and creating dialog include: making "reflecting back" your understanding of some-one's stated values a behavioral norm in decision-making discussions; avoiding jargon by finding fresh ways to express values; using the services of a facilitator to ensure that you have a full, fair, and productive discussion.

When an individual's position is honored and allowed to take root in open dialog, the "health" of the decision-making process is enhanced. Meanings are clarified and participants feel they have been heard and even may be willing to "let go" of certain strong positions that might otherwise impede agreement. Even when full consensus is not possible or is not the goal, comprehensive naming and thorough clarification are necessary for decisions to last.

Weighing: What Do I Think Is the Relative Importance of the Values Involved?

A comprehensive list of interests and values is usually too large to be fully and equally honored. For example, profit, fiduciary responsibility, quality and safety, public reputation, professional autonomy, organizational mission, and increased market share are not entirely compatible. The question thus becomes: If we cannot fully honor all these important interests, which is/are most important? Put another way: If we do nothing else, we must make certain that. . . . (fill in the value).

There are several ways to weigh and prioritize values. Sometimes an "advocacy round" helps. Participants each speak, briefly but strongly, to the value they think is most important. Other techniques include multiple voting, weighted multiple voting, and rank ordering. The rule of thumb is always to use a method that fits the situation. Patterns and agreement begin to emerge, at which point—and only at this point—decision options should be considered.

Deciding: What Action(s) Do I Believe the Most Important Values Warrant?

This entire process is not meant to replace full blown decision-making processes already in use. Rather, it highlights a dimension of decision making that is routinely overlooked in much of decision-making theory and practice—the values base. At the point in any decision-making process where alternative options are generated and considered, each option should immediately be tested against the prioritized list of values. The goal is to develop a decision that is genuinely driven (not just "spun" or superficially rationalized) by the identified top values. The coherence between a decision and its stated reasons must be genuine.

Communicating: How Do I Justify the Decision to Others?

Decision makers may feel, as a matter of course, that they usually work through many of the steps described so far, and they may tout their decisions as strong and sound on that basis. Chances are, however, their communication of decisions and their real reasons frequently leaves something to be desired. People who have a reason to know should be informed about the grounds for the decision. First, who actually made the decision (which is not addressed by leading with, "It was decided that . . .")? How was the decision approached and who was involved? What did the decision makers struggle with? What was most important in making the final decision? What is the decision?

Some decision makers prefer the "bottom-line" approach, starting with the decision and working backwards through the justifying reasons. Others prefer a more contextual or narrative approach that concludes with the decision. The components of a complete report are the same, and the common goal is to explain and justify the decision to stakeholders. Consider the two following "Decision Summary Forms."

> Form No. 1: State the decision in direct, simple language. Be clear who "owns" the decision. (*I/the executive committee . . . have decided to . . .*)
>
> Describe the most important values that "drove" the decision. (*Ultimately, we believe that . . . , . . . , and . . . had to drive our final choice.*)
>
> Directly address the "downside" of the decision, that is, what you do not like about the decision. (*There are some parts of this decision I/we do not like . . .*)

Describe applicable values that could not be honored and indicate the reasoning for your judgment that other values were more important in this situation.

Address any negative impacts of the decision on stakeholders. Pay particular attention to those who were not fully consulted in the decision process.

Form No. 2: How did you approach this decision? (Provide some brief highlights of the decision process, e.g., the steps you took, who was at the table, whom you consulted, the level of time and effort involved.) (*Let me give you a sense of the road we took to get to this decision . . .*)

Be candid about the "downside" of the decision.

Describe applicable values that could not be honored.

Address negative impacts of the decision on stakeholder.

Describe (using everyday language) the values that "drove" the decision.

State the decision in direct, simple language. Be clear who "owns" the decision.

CONCLUSION

Decisions made with integrity are comprehensive, coherent, and transparent (see Table 1a.5). First, the decision maker(s) has made a good faith effort to consider the full range of interests and values (*comprehensive*). Second, the decision is logically grounded in the values held out to be the driving values. That is, the stated basis for the decision genuinely supports the decision (*coherent*). Third, the decision maker communicates the decision to those who deserve to hear about it in a sincere, forthright manner. The decision maker is willing to stand up, be open and accountable to stakeholders by exposing the reasoning for the decision. This requires a willingness to be tested, questioned, and judged by others (*transparent*).

This values-based decision-making process rests on certain important assumptions, observations, and hypotheses. All choices and decisions are driven by values, by what matters. Contemporary business approaches to "ethics" and "integrity" often focus on avoiding wrongdoing or breaking the law. Many decisions, however, are not about right versus wrong, but rather right versus right (competing "goods"). Decisions are effective and enduring when they are based on clearly identified values, are made efficiently, have the resources and support to be fully implemented, and produce positive results that significantly outweigh the negatives. Durable decisions usually follow thorough dialog, consultation, and collaboration.

Table 1a.5: Triangle

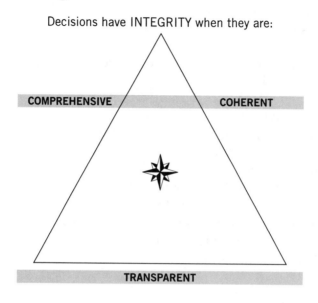

Decisions have INTEGRITY when they are:

COMPREHENSIVE   COHERENT

TRANSPARENT

Isolation is the worst possible counselor.

Miguel de Unamuno, Philosopher, Spain

POSTSCRIPT

The following is a "tool" for a "values analysis on the fly," when time is short but values still must be considered.

1. Come prepared to speak directly to the values dimension of the decision.
   - If you know the issue ahead of time, ascertain what *frame* you bring, what *values* you think are most important, and be prepared to communicate these.
   - Encourage others to think ahead of time about their frames and values.
   - Create the expectation that this kind of "homework" will be done.
2. Commit to a "values round."
   - Ask everyone in the room to explain their frame and values list.

- Avoid jargon and encourage ordinary language that captures the "values in context."
- Listen well and check in with people as they explain their values.
- Record the frames and values where everyone can see and refer to them.
- Weigh these values for relative importance.

3. Return to the values list as appropriate.
- As issues and options are explored, ask: Which value(s) does this choice honor?
- Craft decisions that are genuinely driven by the values that are most important in this situation.

4. Report your values-based decision.
- State the decision and name the values that drove it.
- Acknowledge the values that could not be honored.
- Explain values priorities.

Note

1. Polanyi, M., and H. Prosch. 1975. *Meaning.* Chicago: University of Chicago Press.

CONFLICTING MORAL DEMANDS:
QUAL PLUS HMO

F OR TEN years, Jim Goodrich has been the chief operating officer (COO) of Qual Plus, a successful not-for-profit, staff model–managed care organization in a major metropolitan area on the West Coast that boasts 275,000 members. His organization, in some measure due to Jim's efforts, has been so financially successful that it is about to embark on the construction of a $12 million corporate office complex to house its business activities. As COO, Jim has been responsible for the planning and development of the project, the purchase of the land, and the presentation of the construction proposal to the 12 member board of directors. Following the board's approval, it is the task of the building and grounds committee of the board to select a general contractor and submit the construction contract to the board as a whole for its approval.

The committee established selection criteria for the general contractor that included demonstrated quality of work, ability to meet construction deadlines and work within budget, financial solvency of the firm, and competitive costs. It was also decided that only local firms known to adhere to ethical business practices would be asked to bid on the project.

The requests for bids indicated that all bids must be delivered, sealed, and in hand by noon on 9 December to the COO's office. Bids received after this designated time and not in this designated manner would not be considered. The committee meeting was scheduled for 1:00 p.m. on the ninth to open the bids, review them, and select a general contractor to submit for board approval.

Joe Smith had served on the building and grounds committee for a number of years. Joe was well liked by the other members of the board and had been appointed to this committee because, as the owner of Smith Masonry, he had expert knowledge of construction and related fields.

At the appointed time, the committee met, opened the bids, and began its review. Of the bids received, three appeared to meet all criteria. The costs associated with two of the bids were close. The cost of the third bid, offered by Acme Construction, was considerably higher. Joe was visibly shaken. Jim knew that Acme subcontracted with Joe's firm for masonry work. Because of this, Jim assumed Joe would declare a conflict of interest and abstain when it came time for a vote. Jim did not, however, anticipate what happened next.

As the discussion was about to begin, Joe moved that the committee take a brief 10 minute recess before continuing its deliberations. When the committee reconvened, Joe made a motion that the three contractors who had made the final cut be offered the opportunity to submit a "final" bid in 24 hours. The committee would then reconvene the next day to review these "final" bids. Jim was astonished at the motion and at its immediate support from the rest of the committee and questioned the rationale, legality, and ethical implications of this action. He was told quite simply that since all three finalists were being given the same opportunity, it should not be considered illegal or improper. As for rationale, it was the committee's belief that Acme Construction, who met all of the other criteria, may have inadvertently made an error in calculation that placed its bid so much higher than the other two contractors who were finalists. Joe then spoke on behalf of his motion and indicated that indeed it would be unfair and seem unethical to *not* allow a final bid from a contractor known to be competitive in pricing and who was highly regarded within the building community when the difference in the bid was great enough to appear to be an obvious miscalculation. The question was quickly called and the vote was unanimous to seek "final" bids from the three contractors.

Jim was shocked and angry that the board committee would take action that he believed to be blatantly unethical, if not illegal. And furthermore, that as the responsible administrator for this project, he was expected to concur with their decision, an expectation that he was most uncomfortable with and believed to be in conflict with his responsibility as an administrator. As soon as he was in his office, Jim called the HMO's attorney and reviewed the committee action with him. When asked about the legality of this action, the attorney said he believed it to be a bit unusual but not illegal. Jim was convinced that the attorney was reluctant to explore the matter more fully simply because it was individual board members' actions that were being questioned, rather than board action as a whole.

At this point, Jim knew he had to report the events of the afternoon to Brent, his boss. Brent had been CEO of Qual Plus since its inception 15 years ago and had the unfailing support of the board of directors. Jim liked Brent and his reporting relationship with him had been mutually satisfying. Brent trusted Jim and gave him the latitude to run the operations of the organization. At times Jim felt that Brent might play a little fast and loose with propriety but the issues were always personal ones that did not really affect Jim or the operations of the organization. There had been rumors that Brent had his home remodeled at no cost to him due to the largesse of Joe, and that his automobiles were provided at no cost to him by another board member. He was also known to vacation often in a luxury condo in the Caribbean owned by yet another board member. More disturbing to Jim, however, was the fact that Brent's administrative assistant took care of all of his personal errands and business and was often gone from the office for extended periods of time.

When Jim told Brent of the committee action, Brent dismissed it with a shrug. "It's a board committee, it's their call," he said. Jim persisted and told Brent that he was not comfortable with the committee's actions especially since he was the one expected to execute their decision and that he was going to request an opinion from the Qual Plus ethics committee. Brent appeared agitated at this suggestion and said abruptly, "I would not recommend that, but if you feel you must, go ahead. Just remember, its your job that's on the line here." He then stood up, indicating that the discussion was over.

Jim was disappointed with Brent's reaction. With a mortgage, twin girls in college, a son in high school, and a wife with professional ties to the community, Jim was not prepared to relocate. He doubted strongly if he could match his current salary in another position. Brent and the board had been extremely generous with his compensation package. Jim did not want to jeopardize his position at Qual Plus. On the other hand, he was seriously troubled with his dilemma.

He called the chair of the organization's ethics committee who said that she did not believe this situation fell within the purview of her committee because it was a board action but agreed to poll her committee and get back to Jim with a response by late afternoon. Jim was not surprised when her later call indicated that her committee agreed with her earlier assessment. Jim had come to the conclusion that no one at Qual Plus was ready to take on the board members over this issue. Frustrated, Jim knew that he was expected to "keep his mouth shut" and carry out the wishes of the board committee. But, he also knew that if he did this he would be violating his personal principles and would make himself vulnerable to future expectations of unethical behavior.

ETHICS ISSUES

Conflict of Interest Do Joe's actions here constitute a flagrant conflict of interest? Does Qual Plus have an organizational policy on conflict of interest that specifically provides guidance and direction for governing board members?

Management's Role and Responsibility What is management's role and responsibility in this matter? Specifically, what is the role of the CEO related to actions of governing board members? Have Brent's "special" relationships with board members compromised his position and authority as CEO? Is management's primary responsibility to the governing board or to the organization?

Use of Organizational Resources Is having the administrative assistant perform personal business for the CEO an appropriate use of organizational resources? Is it appropriate for the CEO to accept personal favors of the value of home remodel, luxury cars, and vacations from board members?

Adherence to Organization's Mission Statement, Ethical Standards, and Values Statement Are the actions of the Qual Plus board committee consistent with the organization's mission statement, ethical standards, and values? What about Jim's reaction and the reaction of the CEO?

Adherence to Professional Codes of Ethical Conduct Are the actions here consistent with the codes of conduct as promulgated by the professional organizations and associations representing healthcare executives and managed care organizations?

Organizational Implications What is the role of the Qual Plus ethics committee in this situation? What does it say about the organizational culture if so many staff members appear to find the board committee's action to be acceptable?

Conflicting Moral Demands What is the responsibility of a healthcare executive when he/she is asked to do something that he or she feels is unethical? What is the responsibility of a healthcare executive when the executive observes his or her boss or others acting unethically?

Legal Implications Does the action of the board committee here constitute a violation of the organization's bid process? Is any aspect of this action illegal? What is the responsibility of the HMO's attorney in this case?

Justice and Fairness If not illegal, is this action fair to the other vendors (contractors) who participated in good faith in the bid process as stated in the written request for bids?

DISCUSSION

Conflict of Interest

What is a conflict of interest? Worthley defines a conflict of interest as "any influence, loyalty, or other concern capable of compromising a professional's ability to meet professional obligations."[1] John Boatright uses the definition of "a situation in which two or more interests are legitimately present and competing or conflicting."[2] R. J. Porter reminds us that the oldest definition of all may be the best: "No one can serve two masters, for either he will hate the one and love the other, or he will be devoted to one and despise the other. You cannot serve God and mammon." (Matthew 6:24)[3]

The American College of Healthcare Executives believes that conflict of interest is significant enough to warrant its own section of the organization's *Code of Ethics*. Section III reads that "a conflict of interest may be only a matter of degree, but exists when the healthcare executive: A. Acts to benefit directly or indirectly by using authority or inside information, or allows a friend, relative, or associate to benefit from such authority or information. B. Uses authority or information to make a decision to intentionally affect the organization in an adverse manner."[4] The *Code* goes on to caution healthcare executives to "conduct all personal and professional relationships in such a way that all those affected are assured that management decisions are made in the best interests of the organization and the individuals served by it; to disclose . . . direct or indirect financial or personal interests that pose potential or actual conflicts of interest; to accept no gifts or benefits offered with the express or implied expectation of influencing a management decision; and to inform the appropriate authority . . . of potential or actual conflicts of interest related to appointments or elections to boards or committees inside or outside the healthcare executives' organization."[5]

Conflicts of interest most often involve money. It is an issue when an individual's personal ties could influence his/her professional judgment or when an individual is in a position to influence the business of the organization in ways that could lead to his/her personal gain or that of close family or friends.[6] In some cases individuals may be quick to exercise caution when it comes to their own personal gain but may be lax when it comes to the gain of others in their realm of family and especially of friends. But, the same principle applies.

Hallmarks of conflicts of interest. Worthley has provided healthcare executives with a beneficial and useful summary of his five "hallmarks of conflict of interest." These include:

1. Competing obligations: obligation to organization versus obligation to friend.
2. Appearance standard: the "appearance of impropriety" may be sufficient to compromise the interests of the organization. Would a reasonable person be suspicious of misconduct?
3. Myopia: sometimes people close to the situation do not see it as clearly as those who are not.
4. Fairness: actions taken within a conflict-of-interest situation can be unfair to the legitimate stakeholder. Advantages accrue to one party because a conflict of interest reduces the equal opportunity that would otherwise be available to other parties.
5. Confusion: between official power and unofficial power—informal, unofficial, interactions support confusion.[7]

Of particular relevance in the Qual Plus case here is the value of fairness and how it relates to the other general contractors who have fulfilled the criteria required by the organization's formal bid process. Corporate policies and procedures should be fair, above all, to all parties concerned.

Vinicky, et al. in their essay, "Conflicts of Interest, Conflicting Interests and Interesting Conflicts" referenced by Worthley, point out that conflicts of interest will become more and more common in the ever-changing complexities of a healthcare system in which hospitals and physicians contract for services, in which groups insurers contract with hospitals and physician groups, and where issues of third-party payers, corporation-sponsored research, physician investments, and the like all complicate the relationships involved.[8]

Avoiding conflicts of interest. Recognizing the substance of conflicts of interest, what measures can be taken to avoid their detrimental effects? Academic health centers and universities are especially aware of conflicts of interest associated with physician entrepreneurial activities and academic research, especially when funded by corporations. Some universities require that individuals, upon hiring and periodically thereafter, disclose significant financial, personal, and professional relationships that may be a potential conflict of interest between their academic role and outside interests. Disclosure may be required when:

1. serving as an officer of any entity;
2. investing $25,000 or more in any company whose product is related to the work of the organization;
3. owning 10 percent or more in a partnership or corporation;
4. entering into a consulting arrangement that pays $5,000 or more per year; or
5. agreeing to collaborate in research with any commercial entity.

In addition, it is recommended that individuals should abstain from any decision affecting a company in which they or close family or friends have a substantial interest.[9]

These types of employment agreements do much to prevent issues of conflict of interest from becoming major problems. Some organizations include conflict of interest clauses within senior management contracts and require governing board members to sign disclosure documents upon appointment to the board.

Worthley suggests that questions of conflict of interest can be addressed by structural mechanisms within the organization such as codes of conduct, ethics committees, ethics officers, telephone hotlines, and guidelines for the acceptance of gifts.[10] We must bear in mind, however, that informal realities within each organization have considerable impact upon how business is conducted and what is considered appropriate behavior. Corporate norms, social groups, role modeling, and interpersonal relationships all play a role in helping to determine behaviors. The burden of responsibility for ethical conduct within the organization is placed on the leadership of the organization which is ultimately accountable for the corporate culture.

Professional codes of conduct usually address conflict of interest. The American Hospital Association Management Advisory, "Ethical Conduct for Healthcare Institutions" states:

> Healthcare institutions should have written policies on conflict of interest that apply to officers, governing board members, and medical staff . . . Particular attention should be given to potential conflicts related to referral sources, vendors, competing healthcare services, and investments. These policies should recognize that individuals in decision-making or administrative positions often have duality of interest that may not always present conflicts. But they should provide mechanisms for identifying and addressing dualities when they do exist.[11]

State licensures for professionals may include standards of conduct that address conflict of interest, as well.

Organizational policies and procedures should be written to provide guidance for employees and staff that help them to define and avoid conflict of interest situations. A formal bid process typically embodies this kind of protection for staff and ensures fair and equal treatment to vendors. The process and the selection criteria should be well publicized and bids should be solicited from the broadest range of potential providers. The bids should be sealed and confidential and opened and reviewed simultaneously. Under no circumstances should one vendor know of another's bid. The integrity of the perception of wrongdoing is to be avoided. Rumors of unethical business practices, even if untrue, may damage the reputation of the organization and cause it to lose future business.[12] Improperly disclosing confidential information of one vendor to another could even encourage litigation.

O'Connell suggests that to ensure the integrity of the bid process, a blind consideration of all bids on merit without identifying names could be established. If there is any question of conflict of interest, the individual involved "should remove himself/herself from the process to avoid the perception of conflict of interest, collusion, or rigged bidding."[13]

Clearly, policies, procedures, codes of conduct, and the like will assist the healthcare manager avoid problems associated with conflicts of interest. Just as important is candid, open discussion among coworkers and professional colleagues when questions of conflict of interest arise. This kind of honest dialog can help substantially eradicate any perceptions of wrongdoing before they develop.

Management's Role and Responsibility/Leadership

It is generally accepted that the executive leaders within healthcare organizations are expected to be "servant leaders," that is serving the needs of their organization and its stakeholders. There are times, however, when this leadership style may be problematic. "This becomes a challenge if the demands of the organization push the leader to the point of compromise on personal standards or beliefs."[14] When a board member is using his board appointment to influence his personal financial gain, it presents a "precarious" situation for the CEO.[15] Strong, capable leadership can handle this situation without compromising personal integrity. "Sometimes responsibility to the organization does require personal compromise, but it is important to distinguish between compromising our personal preferences and compromising our personal beliefs and goals."[16] There is also a clear distinction between a CEO's responsibility to the organization and his/her responsibility to a board member. Edwards reminds us that "the executive management of an organization has an obligation to protect the interests of the organization, its owners and the community that outweighs any consideration for an individual board member."[17]

So, what should Brent have done in the case of Qual Plus? An appropriate and ethical approach on the part of a CEO in this situation may have been for the CEO and the board chair to meet and discuss the situation, and then privately meet with the board member in question and review the inappropriateness of his actions related to the bid process. Of course, this approach assumes that the CEO in this case has previously put into place guidelines and codes of conduct for the organization and the board, which include signed documents of conflict of interest disclosures. This approach also assumes that the CEO has been a visible exemplary role model for ethical conduct throughout the organization and the community and has included ethics education as part of the board's orientation and continuing education. Certainly, one might suggest that if these structural mechanisms were in place questionable ethical practices like the one surrounding the Qual Plus bid process would not have occurred.

Further complicating this situation at Qual Plus and Brent's leadership abilities has been his lack of behavior as an effective role model. He dismisses Jim's concerns with little thought. He does not take the situation or Jim's discomfort with it at all seriously and offers no support or willingness to pursue an analysis of the ethical implications of the board committee actions.

Use of Organizational Resources

The CEO's cavalier personal use of organizational resources sends a signal to employees and staff that such "misuse" is okay. He uses his secretary as his personal valet while the organization pays her salary and reaps small benefit from her time "at work." He drives luxury cars and takes frequent Caribbean vacations. He has created an impression of a lavish lifestyle garnered from being an executive for an HMO at a time when "managed care has gained a reputation for being 'cheap'— for trying to spend less at the expense of patient care quality."[18] He has provided fertile ground for the appearance of impropriety and suspicions that there may be questionable business practices that are just not visible. Managed care organizations, like other healthcare institutions, are vulnerable to public scrutiny and accountability because they receive public benefits in the form of tax exemptions. Any suggestion that the operations and the business practices of the organization involve conflict of interest, profit-making, or unethical practices may threaten the organization's tax status.

Executives with reputations for excess have been in trouble with the law, with the government, and with the public. The 1994 indictment of three United Way of America executives for stealing $1 million from the charity and spending much of it on personal luxuries came to light because of lavish indulgences like chauffeurs, first-class hotels, and "cost is no object" vacations.[19] An $8.5 million aircraft, a crew of 13 for four days, and a cost of $200,000 to fly one four-star general home from overseas created quite a scandal for the U.S. Air Force in that same year. The general involved in that case was said to have "a reputation for excess."[20]

In addition to Brent's lavish lifestyle, there is a question concerning the propriety of the gifts and favors he receives from board members. The giving of gifts is a reciprocal act where the recipient is expected to express gratitude in some way, by a subsequent gift or favor or consideration bestowed upon the one giving the gift. In this case, what could the board members presenting these gifts to Brent reasonably expect in return? Of course, the answer here, as any experienced senior-level manager knows, is political considerations and personal favors. The manager may be on dangerous ground because he develops a sense that he is beholden to the gift giver and may be expected to provide favors that compromise his obligations to the organization and to the other board members. This may, in some part, account for Brent's reluctance to challenge the board committee's actions at Qual Plus. Brent's reluctance to challenge the board committee is mirrored by the reluctance of the ethics committee and the attorney representing Qual Plus. The staff and employees within an organization take their cues from the CEO and the role modeling that he/she demonstrates on a day-to-day basis. Such is the power of example. The CEO has the responsibility for establishing an ethical culture within the organization, implementing standards of ethical conduct, educating trustees and staff in these standards, and fulfilling the organization's ethical responsibilities to its community. The CEO must conduct his or her personal and professional life in an ethical manner worthy of emulation. While clinicians may bring their own codes of conduct to the workplace, it is management that must set the tone for how business is conducted, how professionals interact, and how patients and clients are served. Behavioral scientists have proven conclusively that it is the culture of the organization that very quickly teaches newcomers what is acceptable, what is rewarded, and what is frowned upon.

Adherence to Organization's Mission Statement, Ethical Standards, and Values Statement

While an organization must have a code of conduct, clear ethical standards must also be articulated and well understood by all members of the organization. Formal education of staff, trustees, physicians, vendors, and suppliers must ensure that everyone knows the ethical rules governing the organization, and plays by them. Each program decision, resource allocation, personnel practice, corporate policy, etc., whether at the board level or below must be undertaken only after the ethical implications have been examined and found to meet the standards of the organization. In an ethical culture, staff are encouraged to question decisions and probe for the ethics issues that may be present. Forums for discussions and mechanisms for consultation contribute to sound ethical decisions.

A major responsibility of the CEO in the development of an ethical culture is educating trustees. Since trustees are typically community members, often in business, it is especially important that the board have a clear conflict of interest policy. The governing board must mandate that each trustee declare conflicts of interest and abstain from voting whenever decisions of the board would bring business advantages to them, either directly or indirectly. Policies related to competitive bidding procedures must be clear and information held confidential.

Most trustees are aware of their fiduciary responsibilities to the organization. Too often, however, financial decisions may be reached without a full understanding of the ramifications. Trustees have an ethical responsibility to make informed financial decisions and to spend the organization's resources wisely. The healthcare executive must assist trustees in fulfilling this obligation by providing complete information and recommending continuing education when needed.

Information regarding patients, clients, physicians, staff, suppliers, and the organization must be treated as confidential by trustees unless otherwise specified. Frequently, trustees may be called upon by friends or family to provide information that must be kept in confidence. A clear confidentiality policy must be in place and well understood.

Only a few of the areas requiring trustee education are mentioned here. These areas were chosen because of their relevance to the case in point. Roberts and Connors highlight several knowledge requirements for effective governing boards and place ethical decision making high on the list.[21] However, some CEOs do not make board education the priority that they should. Some are not interested in a strong, effective board for fear that it might decrease their own power in spite of the fact that ineffective boards are of little value to their organizations.[22]

Adherence to Professional Codes of Ethical Conduct

The American College of Healthcare Executives has published an "Ethics Self-Assessment" designed to help healthcare executives evaluate their personal responses to ethical questions. Among the many questions included are three that are relevant to the Qual Plus case:

1. I have a system in place for board members to make full disclosure and reveal potential conflicts of interest.
2. I personally disclose and expect board members, staff members, and clinicians to disclose any possible conflicts of interest before pursuing or entering into relationships with potential business partners.
3. I advocate ethical decision making by the board, management team, and medical staff.[23]

These questions are one of several tools intended to guide healthcare executives in developing an ethical corporate culture. The best practices of other healthcare organizations can provide valuable guidance and direction. Two examples immediately come to mind. In the early 1990s, the Presbyterian Healthcare System in Dallas, Texas created a "Code of Business Ethics" and a "Pledge to My Peers" as part of its *Strengthening Our System Culture* Project. Complementing the system's mission, values statements, vision, goals, and expectations, these documents became powerful tools for ensuring an ethical corporate culture.[24]

At Allina Health System the merger of a health plan and a healthcare delivery organization stimulated an ethics framework that guides relationships with patients, health plan members, employer customers, employees, and providers. The framework includes clear ethical principles as a "bedrock for decision-making at all levels" that address stewardship, respect, caring, advocacy, honesty, and confidentiality.[25]

With the advent of compliance programs, the opportunity presented itself to combine the responsibilities of compliance and ethics management within an organization. While a compliance program may address some ethical issues, it is recommended that separate compliance and ethics programs be established that complement one another. Whitley and Heeley caution that conduct that is legal may not be ethical even though to be ethical an organization must comply with legal and ethical mandates.[26]

Carter McNamara provides us with ten benefits of managing ethics in the workplace:

1. Attention to ethics improves society.
2. Ethics programs help maintain a moral course in turbulent times.
3. Ethics programs cultivate teamwork and productivity.
4. Ethics programs support employee growth and meaning.
5. Ethics programs help ensure policies are legal.
6. Ethics programs help avoid criminal acts and help to lower fines if acts occur.
7. Ethics programs help with quality management, strategic planning, and diversity management.
8. Ethics programs promote a strong public image.
9. Ethics programs strengthen organizational culture, improve trust in relationships, support quality of products, and cultivate sensitivity to values.
10. It is the right thing to do.[27]

A paramount responsibility of the leadership in an organization, especially in a healthcare organization whose mission is to serve humanity, is to create a corporate culture where sound ethical decisions are a way of life. Healthcare executives must not forget that "the essence of a profession is that its members commit themselves to a set of standards higher than the morals of the marketplace."[28]

Organizational Implications—Evaluating the Effectiveness of Ethics Committees

Historically, ethics committees and ethics consultants within healthcare organizations were called upon to assist in resolving ethical issues related to end of life, access to treatment, and the like. Typically, the majority of committee members were clinicians and the knotty issues brought to these committees were clinical in nature. Today, " . . . the distinction between bedside and boardroom ethical issues is becoming increasingly blurred" and ethics committees are being required to review their scope and functions and to include organizational and business issues within their purview.[29]

The increased complexities of a healthcare system involved in managed care contracting, mergers and acquisitions, compliance issues, physician investment, and the like demand the attention of ethics committees today. The "business" of healthcare has taken on a new meaning and healthcare relationships have become broader and more varied. Healthcare executives are confronted with more ambiguities, potential for ethical dilemmas, and uncharted waters than ever before. The expansion of ethics committee responsibilities to include organizational issues and to provide advice and counsel to healthcare managers is long overdue. Typically, healthcare managers who may be familiar with the clinical issues may be inexperienced with the business issues they now encounter. If ethics committees do not expand their purpose, they may not be used where the greatest need exists.

Paul Hofmann provides us with a number of additional reasons why ethics committees may be underutilized. Inaccurate perceptions of the committees' role and function, low visibility, and confusion about how to access the committee may be problems. Staff may not know the committee is advisory and its deliberations confidential. If committee membership is strictly clinical, non-clinical staff may be reluctant to use it. The committee may suffer from a lack of leadership, support, or initiative. All of these characteristics can contribute to underutilization.[30]

William Nelson believes that effective ethics committees must have a consensus on purpose, clear guidelines on all functions, and broad and balanced professional representation on the committee that reflects the diversity of the organization and the community. He believes members should be primarily volunteer rather than assigned, and should be "reasoned thinkers regarding ethics."[31]

Whitley and Heeley caution healthcare executives to avoid combining an ethics program with an organization's compliance program because conduct that is legal may not be ethical. An effective "ethics strategy should inspire ethical behavior and encourage integrity."[32]

Evaluating the effectiveness of ethics committees requires attention and administrative support. In order for sound ethical decisions to be made on a daily basis within a healthcare organization, an effective ethics committee that reviews and advises on both clinical and organizational issues must be readily accessible to staff.

For practical strategies on evaluating the effectiveness of ethics committees and useful insights on committee self-assessment, Rebecca

Dobbs provides us with valuable information from her extensive research in this area (see Chapter 2b).

Conflicting Moral Demands

Ethical dilemmas faced by healthcare managers are seldom one-dimensional and are rarely, if ever, under the sole control of a well-meaning manager. By definition, a dilemma is conflicting choices with different consequences, usually undesirable. The conflicting moral demands of one's "boss" and one's conscience is a major challenge for the most ethical of healthcare managers. Clearly, this dilemma is what lies at the heart of the matter in the Qual Plus case.

Apparently, this dilemma is not all that uncommon. In survey results reported by John MacIntyre in 2000, 24 percent of American workers said their employer asked or ordered them to do something they considered unethical. Of those, 445 said they did the unethical deed without objecting.[33] A *USA Today* survey, "The Unethical Worker," reported that as many as 56 percent of workers say coworkers commit ethical infractions.[34] In an employee survey within a New Mexico State government department, 39 percent said they had been asked to do something unethical by one in authority. This survey also "showed that managers have to make it clear that staffers can identify possible wrongdoing without fear of retaliation."[35] A study of Professional Secretaries International reported that as many as 58 percent of those surveyed had been asked to do something unethical by their bosses and had done it for fear of losing their jobs. Infractions ranged from lying, falsifying time sheets, sharing confidential information, removing or destroying damaging information, falsifying expense accounts, and preparing documents with false or misleading information.[36]

So what does one do when asked by one in authority to act unethically? Marilyn Moats Kennedy says it is commendable to stand up for what is right, but before you do, you should calculate the costs and make an informed decision before you act. Most people, she says, cannot afford to stand up for their principles on the job. While encouraging workers to do what is right, she cautions them to recognize that they run the risk of being fired, blackballed, or even wrong.[37]

Indeed, employees facing this dilemma are at great personal risk if they decide to refuse to perform unethical acts, especially as in the Qual Plus case, if those in authority are the CEO and board members who control Jim's job and to some extent his future career. Aside from potentially losing his job, what other considerations must weigh heavily upon Jim's decision? What about his family obligations, the education of children, his wife's ties to the community? Jim believes he would have difficulty matching his current compensation package if he were fired. Is this a valid consideration in his decision making? Is his personal well-being and the well-being of his family separate from morality? How would he explain his termination, if that should occur? What about his references for new employment? Would he be labeled as "not a team player"? Is he the only one who sees anything wrong here? Would all of the parties involved deny any wrongdoing if this were made public? Does Jim have any personal liability if he acts unethically? On the other hand, if Jim acquiesces to the board committee's requests and takes action that he deems unethical, what consequences can he expect? Jim knows that he will have difficulty living with himself if he makes this decision. It will be a terrible blow to his self-esteem. He worries that if he complies with the committee's wishes, he will be expected to abandon his principles in future decisions, in essence, be "held hostage" by this action to whatever unethical murky situations may lie ahead. Most employees simply give in under this kind of pressure and become "organization people." To follow one's conscience and defy authority takes a great deal of courage. David Ewing, retired executive editor of *Harvard Business Review*, says:

> There is very little protection in industry for employees who object to carrying out immoral, unethical, or illegal orders from their superiors. If the employee doesn't like what he or she is asked to do, the remedy is to pack up and leave. This remedy seems to presuppose an ideal economy, where there is another company down the street with openings for jobs just like the one the employee left.[38]

Given all the risks involved, is it easier for senior level managers to defy authority than it is for a secretary or an administrative assistant? Who has more to lose?

Indeed, this is a very gloomy situation, but are there any options for those who find themselves in this predicament?

Richard Nielson says there are interventions that one can employ in such situations. These include:

1. Secretly blowing the whistle within the organization.
2. Quietly blowing the whistle, informing a higher-level manager.
3. Secretly threatening the offender with blowing the whistle.
4. Secretly threatening a responsible manager with blowing the whistle outside the organization.
5. Publicly threatening a responsible manager with blowing the whistle.
6. Sabotaging the implementation of the unethical action.

7. Quietly refraining from implementing the unethical order.
8. Publicly blowing the whistle within the organization.
9. Refusing to implement the unethical action.
10. Refusing to support a cover-up in the event unethical action is detected.
11. Secretly blowing the whistle outside the organization.
12. Publicly blowing the whistle outside of the organization.[39]

It is clear that each of these interventions has its limitations. In order for them to be effective, Nielson reminds us that the employee involved must have information that is complete and accurate. Even then, relationships will be damaged. If the employee's allegations of wrongdoing are false, the organization will be damaged. If the allegations of wrongdoing are true, a "gotcha" culture can be created where employees are looking for evidence of wrongdoing on the part of coworkers in the future. While the above interventions may be effective, they can also be destructive.[40]

Nielson advocates for leadership interventions instead, if at all possible. Leadership interventions require working with key people within the organization to arrive at a consensus that provides an ethical solution. The leader must get all to agree to act in the best interests of the organization. However, not everyone has the leadership skills to accomplish this. Also, it takes time that might not be available and it requires an organizational culture that is open to this kind of dialog.[41]

The federal government recognized the difficulty that employees faced when they were asked to do something unethical or when they observed unethical conduct on the part of their coworkers. In 1991, Congress passed the Federal Sentencing Guidelines for Corporations. The guidelines mandate strict punishment for those convicted of federal crimes and hold that an organization is responsible for the wrongful acts of its employees if the employees are acting in their official capacities. The guidelines include fines for the organizations and jail sentences and/or fines for those involved as well as for managers and executives whether they knew about the illegal actions or not. If the company has an effective ethics and compliance program, penalties may be drastically reduced. Criteria for an effective program include:

1. compliance standards and procedures;
2. oversight by high-level personnel;
3. due care in delegating authority;
4. training programs that communicate ethical standards and ensure compliance;
5. internal auditing and reporting systems;

6. consistent enforcement of standards through disciplinary measures; and
7. measures to prevent reoccurrence of offences.

Under these guidelines, employees are expected to be trained and counseled to act lawfully and ethically. In addition, employees must be able to report suspected violations without fear of reprisal.

Other governmental agencies such as the Environmental Protection Agency, the Department of Health and Human Services, and the Department of Justice's Antitrust Division have developed or are developing model compliance programs, programs for self-reporting, and programs for amnesty. Industry and affinity organizations have begun sharing "best practices" for compliance and ethics training.[42]

In the first two years of the enactment of the Federal Sentencing Guidelines for Organizations, 31 organizations were sentenced and only one had an effective program. Healthcare organizations need to be aware that these guidelines apply to all profit and not-for-profit organizations, associations, corporations, and the like where employees number ten or more.[43]

Tim Barnett reminds us that in addition to the Federal Sentencing Guidelines, employees of most organizations are guaranteed protection against reprisal when they disclose actions that violate federal statues. Title VII of the Civil Rights Act, the Age Discrimination in Employment Act, and the Occupational Safety and Health Act all contain anti-retaliation protection.[44] In his same article, Barnett tells us that a recent review of whistle-blowing incidents showed that "among whistle blowers surveyed, 62% lost their jobs, 18% felt that they were harassed or transferred and 11% had their responsibilities or salaries reduced."[45]

So, while there is some protection out there for those who do not wish to participate in unethical or illegal acts or stand by while they observe others participate, there are still risks involved. Healthcare managers who find themselves in this dilemma must carefully weigh the consequences of their actions and the current and future impact of their actions on them personally as well as on family, colleagues, and those within his/her sphere of influence for whom the manager is a role model.

Notes

1. Worthley, J. A. 1999. *Organizational Ethics in the Compliance Context*. Chicago: Health Administration Press. 153.
2. Boatright, J. R. 1993. *Ethics and Conduct of Business*. Englewood Cliffs, NJ: Prentice-Hall, Inc. 169.

3. Porter, R. J. 1992. "Conflicts of Interest in Research: The Fundamentals." In *Biomedical Research*, edited by R. E. Porter and T. E. Malone. Baltimore, MD: Johns Hopkins University Press. 125–6.

4. American College of Healthcare Executives' *Code of Ethics*. 2000. Section III.

5. Ibid.

6. Association of Academic Health Centers. 1990. "Conflicts of Interest in Academic Health Centers—Policy Paper: A Report by the AHC Task Force on Science Policy." Washington, DC. 6–7.

7. Worthley, 153–54.

8. Worthley, 158.

9. Association of Academic Health Centers, 48–50.

10. Worthley, 154.

11. American Hospital Association Management Advisory. 1992. "Ethical Conduct for Health Care Institutions."

12. Edwards, G. 1996. "Rumors of Unethical Conduct." *Healthcare Executive* (May/June): 48–9.

13. O'Connell, L. J. 1996. "Recognizing Conflicts of Interest." *Healthcare Executive* (May/June): 48–9.

14. Ross, A. 1992. *Cornerstones of Leadership for Healthcare Executives*. Ann Arbor, MI: Health Administration Press. 36.

15. Ibid.

16. Ross, 37.

17. Edwards, 43.

18. Fulton, J. 1999. "The Ethics of Managed Care." *Healthcare Executive* (May/June): 65.

19. Weiner, T. 1994. "United Way's Ex-Chief Indicted in Theft." *New York Times* September 14.

20. Hackeworth, D. 1994. "Big Bird, Bad Move." *Newsweek* December 19, 28–9.

21. Roberts, C. and E. J. Connors. 1998. "Major Challenges Facing Governing Boards of Healthcare Delivery Organizations." *Journal of Healthcare Management* 43(4): 297–301.

22. Kovner, A., R. Ritvo, and T. Holland. 1997. "Board Development in Two Hospitals: Lessons from a Demonstration." *Hospital and Health Services Administration* 42(1): 87–9.

23. American College of Healthcare Executives. 1998. "Ethics Self-Assessment." *Healthcare Executive* (March/April) 45–9.

24. Presbyterian Healthcare System. 1991. "Strengthening Our System Culture." Project. Dallas, Texas.

25. Ehlen, J. and G. Sprenger. 1998. "Ethics and Decision-Making in Healthcare." *Journal of Healthcare Management* 43(3): 220–1.

26. Whitley, L. and G. Heeley. 1998. "Beyond Compliance." *Healthcare Executive* (May/June) 62.

27. McNamara, C. "Complete Guide to Ethics Management: An Ethics Toolkit for Managers." [Online information retrieved 2/06/01]. http://www.mapnp.org/library/ethics/ethxgde.htm

28. Association of Academic Health Centers, 5.

29. Nelson, W. A. 2000. "Evaluating Your Ethics Committees." *Healthcare Executive* (Jan/Feb) 48.

30. Hofmann, P. 2001. "Improving Ethics Committee Effectiveness." *Healthcare Executive* (Jan/Feb) 58–9.

31. Nelson, 48.

32. Whitley and Heeley, 62.

33. MacIntyre, J. 2000. "Facts of Life." *Spirit* (May) 146.

34. Hall, C. and S. Ward. 1995. "The Unethical Worker." *USA Today* October 18 B1.

35. Jodrack, J. 1996. "Survey: Workers Skeptical of Youth Dept Ethics." *Albuquerque Journal* May 8 C3.

36. Kleeman, C. 1996. "Secretaries Face Ethics Dilemma When the Boss Wants Them to Fib." *Albuquerque Journal* May 8 C3.

37. Kleiman, C. 1996. "Can You Afford Your Principles on the Job?" *Albuquerque Journal* May 20 Business Outlook, 11.

38. Worthley, J. A. 1997. *The Ethics of the Ordinary in Healthcare.* Chicago: Health Administration Press. 287.

39. Nielson, R. 1989. "Changing Unethical Organizational Behavior." *The Executive* by The Academy of Management (May) 123–30.

40. Ibid.

41. Ibid.

42. Desio, P. 2001. "An Overview of the United States Sentencing Commission and the Organizational Guidelines." [Online information retrieved 2/6/2001]. http://www.ussc.gov/guidelin.htm

43. Hadden, R. 1994. "Feds Could Jail Boss if Employee Breaks Law." *Jacksonville Business Journal* December 9–15 13.

44. Barnett, T. 1992. "Why Your Company Should Have a Whistle-Blowing Policy." *SAM Advanced Management Journal* 57(4): 37–42.

45. Barnett, 37.

ETHICAL ISSUES IN MANAGED CARE

Richard H. Rubin, M.D.

INTRODUCTION

Over the past 30 years, the field of medical ethics has become increasingly important in both medical education and clinical practice. Manifestations of the increasing role and presence of medical ethics can be found not just in the escalating number of books and journal articles on this topic, but in the percentage of medical schools in which training in medical ethics is now part of the standard curriculum and the growing number of hospitals nationwide in which ethics committees regularly meet to help resolve perceived ethical dilemmas.

The past 30 years has also seen the growth of managed care to where it is now a major factor in the delivery of healthcare in the United States. Although the term "managed care" refers to a rather heterogeneous group of institutions, a feature common to all managed care organizations (MCOs) is a systematic approach to controlling what had been a skyrocketing escalation in the country's healthcare costs during the 1960s, 1970s, and 1980s.

The increasing prominence of both medical ethics and managed care over the past three decades has resulted in, if not a head-on crash, a number of well-publicized collisions between the two. The reason the two have collided has reflected, in large measure, their quite different perspectives of the moral universe and the social good. Medical ethics, undoubtedly influenced by the civil rights movement and the consumer rights movement,[1] has placed great emphasis on patient autonomy— the notion that each patient has a right to be treated with respect and dignity as well as the right to make all decisions related to his/her health care (the goal being an "optimal outcome" as defined by the fully informed individual patient). The focus has thus been on the primacy of the individual patient, and physicians' responsibility to be advocates for their individual patients.

Managed care, on the other hand, has clearly concerned itself with the health of not only individual patients, but the collective health of a defined population, namely the MCO's membership or so-called "medical commons." The question of what should take precedence in the physician's mind-set, the individual patient or the collective "medical commons," is at the crux of many disagreements between physicians and MCO managers. Over the past decade or so, these often wrenching ethical dilemmas have been complicated by the addition of still another element into the equation, the fact that the majority of MCOs are now of the for-profit variety, with a fiduciary responsibility to their shareholders.

Some have proposed that the potential for conflict among these various constituencies (individual patients, the "medical commons," and shareholders) make the for-profit MCO model so ethically suspect as to have no rightful place in the U.S. healthcare system.[2-3] Others, meanwhile, contend that the currently dominant for-profit model is the most realistic and efficient means of achieving one of managed care's most overarching goals, that is, some semblance of ongoing control over the nation's healthcare costs.[4] While this debate rages on, physicians and managers in the managed care setting continue to face ethical challenges in their day-to-day work lives. This chapter is meant to sort out some of these commonly faced ethical dilemmas and to offer useful and practical guidelines for both physicians and managers. It is also meant to provide both physicians and managers with some appreciation of the issues faced by their counterparts and to help each group gain a better understanding of their counterpart's thinking and perspective.

This chapter will address seven questions:

1. What are the relevant principles of medical ethics?
2. What are the relevant principles of business ethics?
3. What ethical issues are commonly faced by physicians practicing in a managed care setting?
4. What ethical issues are commonly faced by managers in the managed care setting?
5. What are the legal ramifications for both physicians and managers in the managed care setting?

6. What ethical guidelines can be offered to physicians practicing in the managed care setting?
7. What ethical guidelines can be offered to managers in the managed care setting?

RELEVANT PRINCIPLES OF MEDICAL ETHICS

The task of medical ethics is to analyze and hopefully resolve ethical dilemmas that arise in medical practice and biomedical research. Medical ethics is not a static, rigid entity; on the contrary, it is a field where disagreements among acknowledged experts are far from uncommon. Much of medical ethics has concerned itself with end-of-life issues and discussions related to medical decision making in the case of incapacitated patients. For the sake of focusing on the issue at hand, however, the following are six principles of medical ethics with special relevance to managed care.

Autonomy

As already alluded to in the introductory section, autonomy refers to 1) a person's right to be fully informed of all pertinent information related to his/her healthcare, and 2) the person's additional right, after being so informed, to choose or refuse among the available treatment options. Autonomy also implies a respect for the dignity and intrinsic worth of each individual person.

Beneficence

Beneficence is the commitment to "do good." It usually refers to the physician's obligation to work for optimal health outcomes for individual patients (although what constitutes an "optimal outcome" in a given situation is a decision which the competent, informed patient will help the physician determine).

Nonmaleficence

The flip side of beneficence is nonmaleficence—the commitment to "do no harm."

Fidelity

Fidelity is the notion that the physician should be faithful and loyal to the individual patient. It also implies that the physician will, if necessary, subordinate his/her own interests to serve the patient's interests.

Veracity

Veracity (or truth telling) refers to the physician's responsibility to be truthful to the individual patient, avoiding deception and disclosing to the patient all information relevant to the patient's health.

Justice

In the realm of healthcare, justice implies that all patients should be treated fairly, without regard to their race, ethnic background, socio-economic status, or educational level. Distributive justice refers to the related notion that the allocation of limited healthcare resources should be determined on a fair and equitable basis.

All of the above principles represent values that most thoughtful members of society would regard as worthwhile. However, even a brief consideration of the principles will reveal how two or more of these principles could easily come into conflict and how two ethically astute physicians might differ in their viewpoints. For example, although practicing physicians typically think in terms of their responsibility to individual patients (including honoring the autonomy of individual patients), a public health physician entrusted to ensure the well-being of a wider community would be more likely to view distributive justice as an overriding ethical principle. The difference in perspective between the practicing physician and the public health physician reflects, in large measure, whom each regards as the major stakeholders affected by his or her decisions. In the case of the practicing physician, the major stakeholders are the individual patients the physician sees on a day-to-day basis. In the case of the public health physician, the major stakeholders are the members of the community as a whole. It is thus common in the real world of medical practice for ethical principles to come into conflict, with one's perspective typically determining which ethical principle is viewed as paramount in a given situation. The same situation is true whether the different perspectives are held by two physicians or a physician and a managed care executive.

RELEVANT PRINCIPLES IN BUSINESS ETHICS

Like medical ethics, business ethics is an example of what has been termed applied ethics, that is, ethics applied to a specific profession or occupation. In addition, business ethics is also a dynamic field where disagreement among acknowledged experts is commonplace. This disagreement may even extend to a fundamental issue such as what the goal of a business should be.

Many would contend that the obvious goal of any business enterprise is to be as financially successful as possible. Assuming the business enterprise is a publicly traded company, a major related goal would be to maximize profits for shareholders. Viewed in this context, the guiding ethical principle for corporate leadership would be, first and foremost, to reward its investors, those who have risked their own capital in the company's interest. In addition, to take this line of reasoning one step further, any deviation from the investor-first principle might well be viewed as unethical, especially if it ran contrary to what shareholders were led to believe.

Others would contend, however, that investors represent only one group of stakeholders that the corporate leadership needs to consider when making decisions. In this view, the needs of other stakeholders are also a rightful part of the equation. Such non-investor stakeholders include consumers, business partners, and employees. This so-called stakeholder model 5 of business ethics is obviously more complex than the investor-first model, and one that many American businesses are now espousing.

In still a third model, the corporate leadership might decide that the business enterprise should take on the additional role of enhancing the social good and allocating a percentage of its resources for that purpose. A number of American companies have followed this route, although they currently represent a relatively small minority of U.S. corporations.[5-6]

The above three models demonstrate the wide spectrum of thinking in the realm of business ethics. Since a major question in managed care, especially the for-profit model of managed care, has been whether healthcare should be considered "just another business." The Woodstock Theological Center, a non-profit research institute, convened a diverse group of executives, healthcare professionals, and ethicists in 1991 to develop a consensus statement of ethical principles pertinent to the business aspects of healthcare. The six core principles formulated by the Woodstock participants are as follows:[1,7]

1. *Compassion and respect for human dignity.* The Woodstock group affirmed that patient care is the primary goal and responsibility of healthcare enterprises. Furthermore, they declared it would be unethical for healthcare providers to exploit the vulnerability of patients in order to enhance the organization's or a professional's income or profits.

2. *Commitment to professional competence.* All healthcare professionals, including physicians, nurses, or healthcare

executives, have an ethical duty to continue their educational efforts and enhance their competence.

3. *Commitment to a spirit of service.* Healthcare professionals have a responsibility to the community they serve as well as to individual patients. This responsibility extends to providing uncompensated or under-compensated care to the poor and needy.

4. *Honesty.* Healthcare professionals and executives have a responsibility to be truthful in their interactions, including their interactions with each other and with patients and families. Medical records should also reflect this commitment to truthfulness and accuracy.

5. *Confidentiality.* Information pertaining to the patient should be shared only with the express permission of the patient or legal guardian, except as required by law.

6. *Good stewardship and careful administration.* Healthcare professionals have an obligation to utilize health resources wisely, carefully weighing the relative costs and benefits of the available treatment options.

It is noteworthy, although perhaps not surprising, that there are major similarities between the principles of medical ethics listed earlier and the Woodstock compendium of ethical principles for those in the business of healthcare. "Compassion and respect for human dignity," for example, clearly resonates with the principles of patient autonomy, beneficence, and nonmaleficence. In addition, the Woodstock group's principles of "commitment to a spirit of service" and "good stewardship and careful administration" both relate to the notion of distributive justice. Finally, it should be noted that just as there was the potential for conflict between several of the principles of medical ethics cited previously, a similar potential for conflict exists even within the Woodstock group's core principles. In the setting of limited healthcare resources and market competition, for example, can the "provision of uncompensated or under-compensated healthcare to the poor and needy" realistically coexist with "good stewardship and careful administration?"

ETHICAL ISSUES FACED BY PHYSICIANS

Before examining ethical dilemmas faced by physicians in the setting of managed care, it might be beneficial to briefly discuss ethical issues faced by physicians in the pre-managed care (fee-for-service) era. Not to discuss this, in fact, might leave the reader with the erroneous impression that ethical dilemmas for physicians only arose when managed care came on the scene, and that is clearly not the case.

As its name implies, in the fee-for-service model of healthcare delivery, physicians were paid a specific fee for performing a specific service, whether that service was an annual physical examination or bypass surgery. Although some older physicians might harken back to the fee-for-service era as the "good old days," it was not free of its own ethical quandaries. For example, distributive justice was a major (if perhaps inadequately considered) problem since those who were indigent and/or uninsured frequently could not afford the physician's fee and, except for charity care, were essentially shut out of the system. In addition, the physician's fidelity to the patient may, at least in some cases, have been compromised in a system where physicians were financially rewarded for providing services that might have been of questionable or only marginal benefit to the patient. Physicians' veracity (truth telling) may also have been less than optimal in the fee-for-service system if, for example, the physician just happened to be a part owner of the laboratory to which patients were referred for a multitude of tests. One wonders whether this information was routinely disclosed to patients. Finally, in retrospect, nonmaleficence (the obligation to "do no harm") may not have been pursued as much as one would have hoped; one wonders how many patients in the fee-for-service system were ultimately harmed by procedures that were recommended for questionable or marginal reasons by physicians and surgeons who benefited financially from performing as many of those procedures as possible.

Unfortunately, ethical dilemmas for physicians appear to be no less common (and some would argue that they are even *more* common) in the setting of managed care. Many of these ethical quandaries are related to one fundamental question: In the managed care system, where should the physician's loyalty ultimately lie, with the individual patient, the "medical commons," or the MCO itself?[8] This fundamental question leads to a number of branching questions: Should the physician engage in the rationing of healthcare at the bedside of an individual patient? How should the physician respond when he/she believes that the patient requires the specific expertise of a consultant not on the MCO's panel of consultants? Under what circumstances should the physician prescribe medications not on the MCO's formulary, medications which might well be more expensive than those listed on the MCO's formulary? How much information related to diagnostic and therapeutic options should the physician disclose to the patient? Finally, how forcefully should the physician "fight" the MCO when the MCO makes a patient care-related decision with which the physician disagrees?

Rationing Care at the Bedside

A heated disagreement currently exits among medical ethicists as to whether physicians should ration care at the bedside of an individual patient. Some would argue that a "new ethic" requires that the physician's level of concern about the "medical commons" be so pervasive as to influence the physician's recommendations to individual patients.[9] Others, however, contend that to act in this manner undermines the very foundation of the patient-physician relationship, that is, the patient's expectation that the physician is serving as the patient's advocate, recommending those diagnostic studies and those therapeutic interventions which the physician feels are in the patient's best interest.[10] After all, how can the patient trust the physician to "do the right thing" on his/her behalf if the physician at the bedside is primarily thinking about the welfare of the "medical commons"? My own view is that physicians should not engage in rationing healthcare at the bedside of individual patients since it violates the physician's ethical responsibility of fidelity, an ethical responsibility which patients have rightfully come to regard as an underlying premise of the entire patient-physician relationship.

However, that is not to say that physicians should ignore the reality that healthcare resources are not infinite. There are at least three ways that physicians can reasonably do this without violating the trust their individual patients have placed in them. First, physicians need to recognize that there is no ethical obligation to provide care that is clearly useless or futile, whether it is prescribing antibiotics for a viral illness or extending the life of a terminally ill patient with prolonged ventilator care. Second, all things being equal, physicians should prescribe the least costly among effective therapies. Why choose an expensive quinolone antibiotic for an uncomplicated urinary tract infection, for example, when the very inexpensive antibiotic trimethoprim-sulfamethoxazole will suffice just as well? Finally, the question of how best to enhance the well-being of the "medical commons" in an environment of limited healthcare resources is clearly a profound and entirely legitimate concern. I would argue that this issue, and the related matter of priority-setting, should be addressed in a careful and ongoing manner at the MCO's highest policy-making level, with thoughtful input from physicians as well as from the MCO's membership.

Choice of Consultants

A common question that arises for primary care physicians in the managed care setting is whether a specialty consultant on the MCO's panel is the optimal consultant for a given patient's clinical condition.

The following two cases illustrate how such issues can be present in everyday practice.

Case 1: A 50-year-old MCO patient with an inguinal (groin) hernia asked his primary care physician to refer him to a "surgeon in Canada" whom he heard had developed a new technique for hernia surgery.

Case 2: A 74-year-old MCO patient with hearing loss and vertigo was diagnosed as having an acoustic neuroma, a relatively rare tumor of the acoustic (ear) nerve. Even though the MCO had contracted with a local neurosurgeon to handle all of the plan's neurosurgical procedures, the MCO's consulting neurologist advised the primary care physician to refer the patient to a nearby tertiary care medical center because the center had much more experience with the required neurosurgical procedure.

In Case 1, the primary care physician did not agree to the patient's request to be referred to the "surgeon in Canada" since the physician knew that the MCO's extremely competent general surgeon was very experienced in performing herniorrhaphy (hernia surgery) and that a high-quality outcome could be anticipated if the MCO's surgeon performed the operation.

In Case 2, however, the physician decided to refer the patient to the tertiary care center for the more specialized type of operation the patient needed. At first the MCO did not approve this referral, but after a series of appeals by the patient, the primary care physician, and the neurology consultant (and after the patient informed the MCO that he had hired an attorney to ensure that his interests were safeguarded), the MCO reversed its initial decision and the patient subsequently underwent successful surgery at the tertiary care center.

It is thus my view that if the physician has good reason to believe that the patient requires special expertise for appropriate management, then the physician has an obligation to pursue the necessary out-of-plan referral with the MCO's administration.

Nonformulary Prescriptions

In many respects, the issue of prescribing nonformulary medications is analogous to the situation just discussed, namely referring the patient to a consultant not on the MCO panel. If the physician is convinced that a nonformulary drug is superior to its counterpart on the MCO's formulary, then the physician should serve as the patient's advocate and prescribe the nonformulary medication, explaining to the MCO's pharmacists and administration why that choice was made. In addition, physicians should work with the MCO's pharmacy committee to modify the MCO's formulary when they believe such action is in the best interest of patient care.

Disclosure of Information

Physicians should adhere to the ethical principle of veracity (truth telling), disclosing to the patient all information pertinent to the patient's care. This includes all relevant diagnostic and therapeutic options, especially since an informed healthcare decision on the patient's part would be unlikely if such information were to be withheld. Physicians should also disclose to the patient all relevant financial arrangements between themselves and the MCO (see below), since patients have a right to know if possible conflicts of interest exist, especially if such conflicts of interest could potentially affect the care they receive.

In addition to their obligation to communicate in a truthful manner with patients and families, physicians also have an obligation to communicate truthfully with MCOs. Physicians should not try to "game the system" by providing MCOs with inaccurate or incomplete information, even when their rationale for doing so is to assist the patient in obtaining MCO approval for requested consultations, prescriptions, or other services.[11]

Challenging the MCO's Decisions

Several of the above scenarios can place the physician in the position of challenging decisions made by the MCO. Without a doubt, this can be an exceedingly uncomfortable position for the physician, that is, between the "rock" of fulfilling one's ethical responsibilities to the patient, and the "hard place" of being in a potentially adversarial relationship with the MCO itself. The latter possibility is hardly a trivial issue. If the physician is a salaried employee of a staff model MCO, for example, the MCO could conceivably fire the physician for not being a "team player." In the more common situation where the physician enters into contracts with a handful of MCOs to ensure an adequate volume of patients, the MCO could decide to terminate its relationship with the physician. Depending on the precise wording of the MCO-physician contract, such termination (known in the trade as "deselection") can often be accomplished with minimal notice and without explanation or due process. Physicians routinely walk a tightrope in the managed care setting, and one which might cause physicians to be less than forceful in their patient advocacy role.

Financial Incentives and Disincentives

Aside from the threat of deselection, there is still another, even more frequently employed instrument which MCOs use to influence physician behavior. Most MCO-physician contracts feature clauses outlining financial incentives, financial disincentives, or both.[12] In essence, financial incentives/disincentives are meant to engage the physician (or physician group) more actively in the MCO's cost-containment efforts by using a "carrot" and/or "stick" approach. Successful cost-containment efforts over the time period in question will result in the physician (or physician group) receiving a monetary bonus. Whereas incurring excessive patient costs will result in money (usually held in escrow) being withheld. If financial incentives/disincentives are modest or are based on the performance of a sizable group of physicians, it is less likely that physicians will be unduly influenced by these arrangements when caring for individual patients. More problematic, however, is the situation where the financial incentive/disincentive is significant and based on the performance of an individual physician or a small group of physicians. Here, the physician's financial interest may be pitted against the patient's interest in a direct and disturbing way, raising the suspicion, if not the reality, of physician misbehavior if the patient believes that his/her care is somehow being compromised.

ETHICAL ISSUES FACED BY MCO MANAGERS

As is the case for physicians who work in the managed care setting, MCO executives face a variety of ethical challenges on an ongoing basis. Some of these ethical dilemmas are analogous to those faced by physicians, whereas others are quite different.

Persuasive Advertising and Selective Marketing

In the world of advertising, veracity is usually not uppermost in the minds of those who produce radio, television, or print media commercials. The entire point of advertising, after all, is to present the product in the best possible light, and if some less-than-flattering details are left out in the process, then so be it. Unfortunately, in the case of MCO advertising, this can result in the prospective MCO member being misled, as when the ad implies that members of the MCO in question can see whichever specialist they please.[13] It is then left to the primary care physician to "educate" the new MCO member as to how the plan actually works, including the fact that the member typically has to see the "gatekeeping" primary care physician first before a specialty referral can be made as well as the related fact that the MCO member is usually restricted to seeing those consultants on the MCO's panel.

An issue closely related to advertising is marketing. From a "bottom-line" business perspective, it is clearly in the MCO's interest to have a younger, healthier membership than an older, sicker one. Some MCOs have been known to direct their marketing efforts to effectively exclude those members of the community who are most frail or infirm, that is, by holding sign-ups for seniors at dances or movie screenings, events unlikely to be attended by the bedridden, the housebound, or those requiring walkers or wheelchairs. Such selective marketing aimed at attracting the healthiest (and least costly) prospective members has been termed "cherry picking." Although less-than-fully-truthful advertising and selective marketing might be accepted behavior in most businesses, from an ethical perspective, healthcare organizations should refrain from engaging in such practices.

Disclosure of Information

Honesty should be the rule for MCOs not only when dealing with prospective members but also when dealing with those already enrolled in the plan. Patients should have a right to be informed of all pertinent diagnostic and therapeutic options related to their healthcare and have the right to be informed of all financial arrangements between the MCO and its physicians (including incentives and disincentives) that could potentially affect patient care. "Gag rules," where physicians are instructed to withhold such information from patients, should be prohibited.

Financial Incentives/Disincentives

It is not enough for MCOs (and physicians) to simply disclose information pertaining to financial incentives and disincentives. From an ethical standpoint, it is important that such incentives/disincentives be based on the performance of a sizable group of physicians and not be of such magnitude as to place the physician's personal financial interests in direct conflict with the interests of the individual patient under his/her care.

Ensuring Quality

Although it is the duty of each individual healthcare professional to maintain a high level of expertise and competence, it is an overriding responsibility of the MCO to make sure that its membership is receiving high-caliber medical care. From an organizational standpoint, this can be accomplished in several ways:

1. Contracting only with well-trained and suitably credentialed primary care physicians and specialty consultants who are highly regarded in the local or regional medical community.
2. Working with physicians to establish diagnostic and therapeutic guidelines that are evidence-based, especially for commonly encountered conditions.
3. Soliciting thoughtful physician and pharmacist input when developing the MCO's drug formulary, with a periodic review process so the formulary can be kept up-to-date.
4. Providing performance-based feedback to physicians using a carefully conducted and accurate profiling system, again soliciting physician input in the profiling process.
5. Using patient satisfaction measures as an additional means to evaluate physician performance.

Appeal Procedures

The MCO realistically needs to recognize that either patients or physicians, acting in good faith, may on occasion disagree with the MCO's decisions, especially those related to patient care issues. MCOs need to have a clearly outlined appeal procedure in place. This appeal protocol should be logical, reasonable, and fair, and should not be biased against individual patients in their attempt to have their grievances addressed. This is especially true when questions arise as to whether a particular innovative or experimental therapy is covered by the MCO, since the reality is that medicine is an ever-changing field. In addition, it must be clear that the MCO will never act in a punitive fashion or "take retribution" against either patients or physicians who challenge the MCO's decisions or who otherwise participate in the appeal process.

Confidentiality

Like any other healthcare organization, MCOs need to have systems in place to carefully protect patient confidentiality.

Allocation of Resources

Since healthcare resources are finite and it is understood that MCOs must remain economically competitive in a market economy, priorities in allocating healthcare resources need to be established. MCOs should pursue these allocation decisions in an open manner, with input from physicians and the MCO's membership.

Fostering the Social Good

With the current dominance of the for-profit MCO model, the U.S. healthcare system is currently experiencing difficulty financing several domains that may be considered under the general heading of "the social good." These include 1) medical education (and the training of future healthcare professionals), 2) biomedical research, and 3) the care of the uninsured, who currently number over 40 million Americans. The question has been posed as to what role MCOs (including for-profit MCOs) should play in addressing such social concerns. The responsibility of healthcare organizations to promote the social good is not merely an issue raised by "ivory-tower" ethicists. The *Code of Ethics* of the American College of Healthcare Executives, for example, includes the following statements:[14] "The healthcare executive shall work to identify and meet the healthcare needs of the community . . . work to ensure that all people have reasonable access to healthcare services . . . [and] consider the short-term and long-term impact of management decisions on both the community and on society."

LEGAL RAMIFICATIONS FOR PHYSICIANS AND MANAGERS

Ideally, ethical guidelines alone should suffice in causing physicians and MCO managers alike to "do the right thing." At a certain point, however, inappropriate behavior crosses a line in the sand, and becomes not only ethically suspect but also legally negligent.

A landmark and still very illustrative case in the annals of managed care case law is *Wickline v. California.* Ms. Wickline was admitted to a hospital in California in the late 1970s for a peripheral vascular procedure. Following that procedure, her physicians recommended an additional eight days in the hospital for post-procedure care and observation. Ms. Wickline's insurer was MediCal (California's Medicaid program) and MediCal denied Ms. Wickline's physicians' request for eight days additional hospitalization, approving a four-day stay instead. At the end of four days Ms. Wickline was discharged, and unfortunately she subsequently developed complications that necessitated readmission and eventual amputation of her leg. Ms. Wickline did not sue her physicians, whom she regarded as her advocates, but instead sued MediCal, whom she blamed for the abbreviated initial hospital stay. At a lower court level, Ms. Wickline won her suit and was awarded several hundred thousand dollars. MediCal appealed that decision, however, and the Appellate Court, in a 1986 ruling, reversed the lower court's decision. The ruling of the Appellate Court was noteworthy in two respects, as outlined in the following paragraphs:[15]

Third party payers . . . can be held legally accountable when medically inappropriate decisions result from defects in the design or implementation of cost containment mechanisms as, for example, when appeals made on a patient's behalf for medical . . . care are arbitrarily ignored or unreasonably disregarded or overridden.

However, a physician who complies without protest with the limitations imposed by a third party payer, when his medical judgment dictates otherwise, cannot avoid his ultimate responsibility for his patient's care. He cannot point to the healthcare payer as the liability scapegoat when the consequences of his own . . . medical decisions go sour.

The first paragraph indicated that a third-party payer, be it an MCO or a government program like Medicaid, could be sued if its cost-containment policy resulted in medical harm, especially if the treating physician's legitimate objections were arbitrarily ignored or overridden. The second paragraph was clearly aimed at physicians working in a managed care setting and emphasized that the physician's ultimate obligation was to the individual patient and not passive acceptance of the third-party payer's cost-containment policies.

Since *Wickline v. California*, there have been a number of other cases (e.g., *Boyd v. Epstein, Hand v. Tavera,* and *Fox v. Health Net of California*) related to the legal liability of physicians in the managed care setting and/or the legal liability of MCOs.[16–17] Although each of these cases is a bit different, the common thread seems to be that adverse patient outcomes due to cost-containment policies can place the physician and/or the MCO at legal risk. In addition, MCO executives need to be aware of yet another case (*McClellan v. Health Maintenance Organization of Pennsylvania*) in which the court ruled that the MCO in question had an obligation to select and retain only competent physicians. Of note, despite the cases cited above, MCOs have been relatively protected from being sued in state courts for medical negligence because of the 1974 Employment Retirement Income Security Act (ERISA). The purpose of ERISA was to prohibit state regulation of employee pension plans and other employee benefit plans, including health benefit plans.[18] Since most Americans enrolled in MCOs are enrolled through their employer, ERISA has effectively barred most MCO enrollees from suing their MCO for medical negligence in state courts (although it has not prevented patients from suing their MCO physicians in state courts). In their recent (June 2000) decision in the case of *Pegram v. Herdrich*, the U.S. Supreme Court ruled, in essence, to uphold ERISA, continuing MCOs' immunity from medical liability, at least in many of the situations commonly encountered.[19] At the time of this writing, the issue of whether ERISA should be overturned or amended remains the subject of ongoing and intense political debate. ERISA's future will likely be decided in Congress, with the eventual outcome still uncertain.

RECOMMENDATIONS FOR PHYSICIANS PRACTICING IN THE MANAGED CARE SETTING

In the course of their practice in the managed care setting, physicians should consider the following recommendations:[20–21]

1. The physician-patient relationship is the cornerstone of the practice of medicine and physicians should view their primary obligation as the provision of humane, high-quality care to their individual patients.

2. Physicians are not obligated to provide care that is clearly useless or futile. In addition, physicians have a responsibility to choose among the least costly of effective therapies.

3. Any decisions regarding the allocation of healthcare resources should be made on a broad policy-making level and not at the bedside of individual patients. Physicians have a responsibility to participate in these resource allocation decisions, keeping in mind the ethical principle of distributive justice.

4. Physicians should be truthful in their dealings with patients and families. All information that might affect patient care should be disclosed. Such information includes (a) relevant diagnostic and therapeutic options, and (b) all physician-MCO financial relationships that might impact patient care.

5. Physicians should be truthful in their dealing with MCO management, refraining from attempts to "game the system."

6. If they exist at all, financial incentives and disincentives should be limited in magnitude and should ideally be based on the performance of a sizable group of physicians rather than that of a single physician or a small group of physicians. The physician's personal interest should never result in the withholding of care that is medically necessary or medically advisable.

7. Physicians have an obligation to maintain their professional competence and seek appropriate consultation for patient care issues outside their realm of expertise.

8. Physicians should serve as advocates for a system of healthcare that (a) is based on humaneness, high-quality care, and optimal outcomes for patients, and (b) does not place restrictions on access to medical care that is necessary or advisable.

RECOMMENDATIONS FOR MCO MANAGERS

In many respects, recommendations for MCO managers parallel those made for MCO physicians. For example, recommendations regarding truth telling, the fair and equitable allocation of healthcare resources, and the need for financial incentives/disincentives that are modest at most are germane both to physicians and to MCO executives.

Additional recommendations for MCO managers include:

1. Refraining from engaging in misleading advertising or selective marketing, no matter how great the temptation.
2. Establishing and maintaining systems within the MCO aimed at protecting patient confidentiality.
3. Ensuring a high quality of patient care by (a) selecting and retaining only high-caliber healthcare professionals, (b) working with physicians to establish diagnostic and therapeutics guidelines that are evidence-based, and (c) providing performance-based feedback to physicians that is meaningful and accurate.
4. Establishing appeal procedures that are fair and free of punitive overtones.
5. Carefully considering how the organization might contribute to the social good, including medical education, medical research, and the care of the indigent or uninsured.

A BLUEPRINT FOR THE FUTURE: THE TAVISTOCK PRINCIPLES (A WORK IN PROGRESS)

Although there is considerable overlap between the recommendations offered to physicians and those offered to MCO managers, the current perception is that each constituency within the healthcare universe (be they physicians, MCO executives, or others) tend to view healthcare issues through their own particular lens, a fact which often seems to hamper meaningful discussion and interdisciplinary cooperation.

In 1999, a group of interested parties, including physicians, nurses, healthcare executives, economists, and ethicists, convened to develop a set of mutually agreed upon ethical principles. The group, called the Tavistock group since they initially met near Tavistock Square in London, proposed the following seven principles:[22]

- *Rights.* People have a right to health and healthcare.
- *Balance.* Care of individual patients is central, but the health of populations should also be our concern.

- *Comprehensiveness.* In addition to treating illness, we have an obligation to ease suffering, minimize disability, prevent disease, and promote health.
- *Cooperation.* Healthcare succeeds only if we cooperate with those we serve, each other, and those in other sectors.
- *Improvement.* Improving healthcare is a serious and continuing responsibility.
- *Safety.* Do no harm.
- *Openness.* Being open, honest, and trustworthy is vital in healthcare.

The Tavistock principles are similar in spirit to the principles outlined by the Woodstock group nearly a decade earlier. It is reassuring to contemplate that the tone of shared values and productive cooperation embodied in both sets of principles might one day replace the rancor and divisiveness that has all too often characterized the U.S. healthcare system in the recent past. Only time will tell if the for-profit MCO model will be able to adhere to these principles while simultaneously generating the level of profits that investors in other businesses typically expect. However, no matter what model of healthcare delivery prevails in the future, it remains incumbent on healthcare professionals of all stripes and at every level to make sure that the ethical underpinnings of patient care are honored. Otherwise, the public has every right to become disenchanted with healthcare professionals and healthcare institutions alike, and we should not be surprised when it does.

Notes

1. Joint Commission on Accreditation of Healthcare Organizations. 1998. *Ethical Issues and Patient Rights.* Oakbrook Terrace, IL: JCAHO.

2. Pellegrino, E. D. 1999. "The Commodification of Medical and Healthcare: The Moral Consequences of a Paradigm Shift from a Professional to a Market Ethic." *Journal of Medicine and Philosophy* 24(3): 243–66.

3. Woolhandler, S., and D. U. Himmelstein. 1996. "When Money is the Mission — The High Cost of Investor-Owned Care." *New England Journal of Medicine* (341): 444–6.

4. Hasan, M. 1996. "Let's End the Non-Profit Charade." *New England Journal of Medicine* (334): 1055–7.

5. Wong, K. L. 1998. *Medicine and the Marketplace.* Notre Dame, IN: University of Notre Dame Press.

6. Fletcher, R. H. 1999. "Who is Responsible For The Common Good in a Competitive Market?" *Journal of the American Medical Association* (282): 1127–8.

7. Woodstock Theological Center. *Ethical Considerations for the Business Aspects of Healthcare.* Washington, DC: Georgetown University Press.

8. Abrams, F. R. 1986. "Patient Advocate or Secret Agent?" *Journal of the American Medical Association* (256): 1784–5.

9. Hall, M.A. and R.A. Berenson. 1998. "Ethical Practice in Managed Care: a Dose of Realism." *Annals of Internal Medicine* (128): 395–402.

10. Kassirer, J. P. 1998. "Managing Care—Should We Adopt a New Ethic? *New England Journal of Medicine* (339): 397–8.

11. Freeman, V. G., S.S. Rathore, K. P. Weinfurt, K. A. Schulman, and D. P. Sulmasy. 1999. "Lying For Patients: Physician Deception of Third-Party Payers." *Archives of Internal Medicine* 159 (19): 2263–70.

12. Hillman, A. L. 1990. "Health Maintenance Organizations, Financial Incentives, and Physicians' Judgments." *Annals of Internal Medicine* 112 (12): 891–3.

13. Brett, A. S. 1992. "The Case Against Persuasive Advertising by Health Maintenance Organizations." *New England Journal of Medicine* 326 (20):1353–7.

14. Hall, R. T. 2000. *An Introduction to Healthcare Organizational Ethics.* New York: Oxford University Press.

15. *Wickline v California*, 226 *Cal. Rptr.* 661 (Cal. App. 2 Dist., 1986).

16. Gosfield, A. G. 1995. "The Legal Subtext of the Managed Care Environment: A Practitioner's Perspective." *Journal of Law, Medicine & Ethics* 23 (3): 230–5.

17. Moskowitz, E. H. 1998. "Medical Responsibility and Legal Liability in Managed Care." *Journal of the American Geriatrics Society* 46 (3): 373–7.

18. Mariner, W. K. 1996. "State Regulation of Managed Care and the Employee Retirement Income Security Act." *New England Journal of Medicine* 335 (26): 1986–90.

19. Mariner, W.K. 2000. "What Recourse?—Liability For Managed Care Decisions and the Employee Retirement Income Security Act." *New England Journal of Medicine* 343 (8): 592–6.

20. Council on Ethical and Judicial Affairs, American Medical Association. "Ethical Issues in Managed Care." *Journal of the American Medical Association* 273 (4): 330–5.

21. Rubin, R. H. 1999. *Gatekeepers and Gatekeeping in Managed Care: Financial, Legal and Ethical Issues* edited by D.A. Bennahum. Cleveland, OH: Pilgrim Press.

22. Davidoff, F. 2000. "Changing the Subject: Ethical Principles for Everyone in Healthcare." *Annals of Internal Medicine* 133 (5): 386–9.

EVALUATING HEALTHCARE ETHICS COMMITTEES

Rebecca A. Dobbs, R.N., Ph.D., FACHE

INTRODUCTION

The healthcare system in the United States has undergone radical changes in its structure, delivery and financing of services, and its role in society. The current environment is characterized by an increased awareness of patient rights and responsibilities, increased treatment choices, significant advances in biomedical technology, still higher costs, and the powerful influence of insurers in healthcare delivery and decision making.[1] This era also depicts the broad changes occurring in social values and public expectations, not just the mechanics of healthcare delivery and financing. Newly raised ethical concerns stemming from resource allocation issues (e.g., rationing of care), scientific and technological advancements (e.g., human genetics), moral duplicity (e.g., assisted suicide), evolving financial arrangements (e.g., conflicts of interest), and increased attention to quality and accountability pose new challenges for healthcare institutions and professionals.[2-8] Societal norms and expectations have a significant impact on professional behavior within healthcare. Any change to these norms and expectations raises fundamental questions and issues regarding public policy and the future nature of health services. Questions regarding access and accountability will surface due to the high value placed on universal access and individual freedom. Technologies developed for the treatment, prevention, and early detection of medical conditions will also raise new ethical questions about who will have access to these advancements, who will control their use and distribution, and what effect those decisions will have on already strained provider-patient relationships.[9] Coupled with an increase in external regulation and bureaucracy in healthcare, continuing evolution of the provider-patient relationship, more limited patient choices, and the family's expanded role in decision making as a result of an aging population,[10] healthcare organizations will find it increasingly important to have a formalized ethics program in place.

Many healthcare organizations have already recognized the need for a comprehensive ethics program—one that goes beyond the Joint Commission on Accreditation of Healthcare Organizations (Joint Commission) standard which merely requires that a mechanism be in place for dealing with ethical concerns arising in patient care.[11] Historically, such "mechanisms" have taken a variety of forms. Some healthcare organizations have chosen to use individual ethics consultants and bioethicists, some have written extensive ethics policies and procedures to be carried out by an existing organizational committee or entity, and still others have formed ethics committees dedicated to the task of dealing with clinical ethics issues as they arise.

In recent times, many organizations have created positions for ethics officers or compliance officers to monitor the organization's adherence to ethical standards. Few, however, have ventured into the realm of a fully integrated healthcare ethics program—one that monitors the ethical climate of the organization, proactively addresses potential ethical issues, aggressively manages ethical discourse in the clinical as well as the organizational context, critically evaluates its overall effectiveness, and takes action to change the organization's ethical culture and processes. Efforts to do so thus far have primarily been characterized by the merging of existing organizational entities (e.g., compliance, accreditation, quality assurance, risk management, and clinical ethics) under a new organizational title. Therefore, until such a fully integrated healthcare ethics program matures enough to meet the growing ethical needs of healthcare organizations, the healthcare ethics committee (HEC) will most likely remain the primary vehicle for the fielding of ethical issues within most healthcare organizations. However, the healthcare ethics committee is also undergoing dramatic changes as it is pressured to take on the task of responding to an increasing number of organizational ethics concerns that cannot be disentangled from the purely clinical ones.

The U.S. healthcare system continues to face demands for accountability as evidenced by the passion with which many healthcare organizations have adopted performance assessment and improvement approaches. Healthcare programs are increasingly expected to justify their existence, document their operations, and strategically plan future activities.[12] Healthcare ethics committees are no longer in their infancy but are, in fact, powerful influences in healthcare decision making. Formalized requirements for performance assessment and improvement have not been extended to HEC functions and processes, nor do widely publicized and accepted performance standards exist to guide HEC activities. Still, it is not unreasonable to expect an increased level of scrutiny and accountability with respect to healthcare ethics committees.

HEC FUNCTIONS

Cranford and Doudera and other notable authors describe the work of HECs as consisting of three primary functions, education, policy development, and case consultation.[13]

Education

The ethics education function serves three principal audiences: the ethics committee itself, the staff within the organization, and the community at large. Ethics committee member education is widely accepted as a major priority. Educational initiatives frequently focus on ethical theories and principles, medical-legal issues, the application of ethical theories and principles to ethics policy/guideline development and ethics review/consultation, committee functions and obligations, group processes, and communication skills. Educational goals may vary greatly depending on the HEC's mission and objectives, committee member needs, organizational setting, and available resources. Ethics education is also provided within the organization and frequently focuses on improving the staff's understanding of general bioethical and medical-legal issues as they relate to medical treatment and patient care activities. Topics often include current issues in bioethics and information on institutional policies and procedures. Community education efforts focus on stakeholders that exist beyond the confines of institutional boundaries. Educational opportunities within the community can be addressed by providing local workshops on selected topics, conducting focus groups designed to share information and solicit input for policy development and revision, working with university faculty on curriculum development, working with legislators to develop new legislation, and testifying before legislative bodies. The success of community education depends largely on adequately identifying the needs and interests of the target audience and planning educational opportunities accordingly.[14–16]

Policy Development

The ethics policy/guideline function addresses those committee activities related to the development, implementation, review, revision, and compliance assessment of ethics policies and guidelines. Ethics policies tend to define ethical boundaries or establish standards within which specific activities must occur; whereas, ethics guidelines tend to be more flexible and less prescriptive by suggesting options or alternatives to a given ethical situation. The level of HEC involvement in the ethics policy/guideline process varies among healthcare organizations. Some committees have direct involvement in ethics policy/guideline activities while others take on more of a consultative role. Most HECs write policies/guidelines on well-documented topics in which there is broad societal consensus, but some HECs are venturing out into relatively uncharted waters by developing policies/guidelines on clinical issues such as futile care and organizational issues such as resource allocation.[17] The degree of HEC involvement in ethics policy/guideline development is determined largely by organizational culture, the composition and maturity of the committee, and its relationship within the organization and community.

Case Consultation

Ethics review/consultation is performed primarily to assist healthcare professionals, patients, and families/surrogates in sorting out treatment options, making informed decisions, or resolving conflicts. An *ethics review* is generally performed retrospectively to analyze situations in which an ethical concern or issue has been raised. An ethics review can have a positive effect on future situations presenting a similar issue, but its timing prevents it from having any impact on the situation being studied. An ethics review can also be performed proactively in a hypothetical setting which can be particularly helpful for HECs and organizations in working through ethical dilemmas before they occur. It can also provide useful inputs to the development, review, and revision of ethics policies/guidelines. An *ethics consultation*, on the other hand, generally refers to the concurrent analysis of an ethical concern or issue in which the parties involved interact to resolve the ethical dilemma. An ethics consultation can be performed using the whole committee approach, a consultation team, or individual member/ consultant.[18-19] An HEC may elect to use a variety of formats (such as the medical model, legal model, or educational model) for guiding an ethics review/consultation. The *medical model* emphasizes the medical expertise of physicians, nurses, and usually a chaplain in addressing clinical matters. The *legal model* treats the ethics review/consultation as a type of hearing in which input is sought from the parties involved and attention is given to issues of due process. The *educational model* emphasizes the importance of a multidisciplinary approach in exploring the various ethical dimensions of a given situation. Selection of an appropriate model for ethics review/consultation is based largely on the specific ethical issues and the special concerns of those involved.[20]

To these three widely accepted HEC functions, Dobbs added a fourth function—HEC administration/management.[21] The HEC administration/management function addresses activities related to infrastructure, relationship within the organization, strategic planning, committee composition, membership criteria, resource allocation, and performance evaluation. Healthcare ethics committees across the country vary greatly in mission, structure, relationship within the organization, scope of activities performed, and formality of internal processes. Little has been written in the literature regarding HEC administration/management. Thus, HEC administration/management remains one of the most widely varied of the recognized HEC functions.

Bioethics literature confirms the importance of and ongoing need for HEC evaluation. Ross et al. suggest that evaluation is necessary, in part, to enhance HEC credibility and to justify the commitment of increasingly scarce institutional resources.[22] Dobbs points out that information obtained from the HEC evaluation process can be used to (a) identify areas for improvement, (b) prioritize improvement activities, (c) assist in the strategic planning process, (d) plan resource requirements, (e) provide baseline data for future evaluation and benchmarking activities, and/or (f) document activities for internal management reviews and external accreditation surveys.[23] Even though many agree that critical self-assessment of HEC processes demonstrates an organization's commitment to quality healthcare and attention to societal needs and concerns, there is no consensus on which approach is most suitable for conducting such an evaluation.

HEC EVALUATION STRATEGIES

Evaluation strategies commonly used to assess healthcare functions or programs include program evaluation, internal evaluation, and self-assessment. Program evaluation provides a highly structured analysis of program elements and activities by an external source. Internal evaluation provides an organizational perspective of a program's interrelated components and functions as measured by other organizational members. Self-assessment provides an intimate evaluation of a program by those who are directly responsible for its planning, execution, and management.

Program Evaluation

Program evaluation is concerned with the value of a particular program or program elements. According to Sechrest and Figueredo, program evaluation is a process for deciding the worth of various activities within which any number of methods can be used.[24] Program evaluation can be classified as either formative (process-oriented) or summative (outcome-oriented) depending on the type of information produced and how the information is used.[25]

Formative evaluation assesses the process by which the program conducts its activities and is designed to improve the program and its management.[26-27] A formative approach has certain advantages: (a) the general ease with which practitioners can develop performance standards and assessment criteria, and (b) even when not fully validated, the standards and criteria can serve as interim measures of acceptable performance. The major disadvantages to a formative approach are that it may actually encourage dogmatism and perpetuate potential errors in what is determined to be acceptable performance.[28]

Summative evaluation focuses on the long-term effects of a program: its end-product, how well the program is functioning, and whether it has had any impact on given indicators of performance. A summative approach also has certain advantages, in that it (a) tends to discourage dogmatism, (b) reflects the contributions of all practitioners, and (c) provides a more direct assessment of the practitioner-customer relationship when customer satisfaction measures are included. Disadvantages of the summative approach include (a) the difficulty with which practitioners are able to specify outcomes of optimal performance, (b) the ethical issue associated with waiting for adverse outcome trends to emerge before taking action, and (c) the difficulty in drawing pertinent conclusions when outcomes are assessed without evaluating the related processes.[29]

Veney and Kaluzny view program evaluation as an integrated process of collecting and analyzing data using various scientific methods to determine the relevance, progress, efficiency, effectiveness, and impact of program activities. They describe five approaches to program evaluation: monitoring, case studies, survey research, trend analysis, and experimental design.[30]

Monitoring is concerned with program progress and improvement and involves the comparison between program expectations and actual results. Even though some researchers consider monitoring to be mundane or nonscientific, Veney and Kaluzny consider it a necessary component of evaluation—particularly important to formative evaluation and critical to the evaluation of progress and continuous improvement.

Case studies tend to rely more on the ingenuity, insight, and experience of the researcher than other evaluation strategies utilizing more rigorous methods such as sampling and statistical techniques. Even though they may be primarily qualitative in nature, case studies frequently employ a variety of quantitative data collection and analysis techniques.

Survey research has become a common evaluation strategy (particularly in the summative evaluation of programs) and is primarily either descriptive or analytic in nature. Descriptive surveys are used to produce an accurate depiction of the phenomenon being studied by describing a problem that requires some type of program activity, describing the program from the perspective of providers or participants, or describing results of the program from the perspective of the providers or participants. Analytic surveys are used to describe relationships between different aspects of the phenomenon by determining whether program participants having different types of characteristics view a program more or less favorably, or by determining whether there is some differential effect of the program on participants having certain characteristics.

Trend analysis is an evaluation strategy for examining tendencies in performance indicators over time. It can be done in conjunction with monitoring to determine whether the introduction of a particular program can actually be viewed as having a causal connection to changes in the condition that the program was established to influence.

Experimental design is the most powerful program evaluation approach. It can be a complex undertaking even though the basic pattern is relatively simple: the state of a system is observed at a given point in time, an experimental variable is introduced, and the state of the system is observed again to determine the effect of the variable on the system. Some experimental designs may be too complex for healthcare settings. However, those that appear to be feasible and appropriate include: pretest/posttest design, pretest/posttest with a control/comparison group design, multiple group pretest/posttest design, and posttest only design.

Veney and Kaluzny and Donabedian do not favor one evaluation approach over the other; nor do they imply that either the formative or summative approach should be used exclusively. Rather, they contend that a well-designed program evaluation may require a combination of approaches reflective of the nature of the information to be obtained and other requirements of the situation.[31,32]

Internal Evaluation

Another evaluation strategy applicable to healthcare settings is internal evaluation. Performed by persons within the group or organization under study, internal evaluation examines the organization as a set of interrelated components and functions. Data obtained from internal evaluation activities can assist the healthcare organization in: (a) preparing for compliance or accreditation reviews, (b) meeting internal and external reporting requirements, (c) identifying and documenting client/customer needs, (d) describing programs and services, (e) identifying program strengths and weaknesses, (f) collecting data for establishing program priorities, (g) planning budgets, (h) obtaining and maintaining financial support, and (i) relating to external customer groups. Since internal evaluation is a proactive approach that focuses on internal regulation and control, potential problems can be identified more quickly.[33–34]

Self-Assessment

Social values in the twenty-first century call for interdisciplinary team building, trust, responsibility, and accountability within healthcare organizations. Self-assessment is a process by which a healthcare organization or entity within the organization evaluates itself to systematically monitor performance against established standards.[35–36] Wilson and Pearson describe three forms of self-assessment: compliance, compliance plus effectiveness, and performance. Compliance self-assessments are generally performed on a routine, periodic basis in anticipation of an upcoming external evaluation. Compliance self-assessments that include an evaluation of effectiveness are often performed to identify system improvements. Performance-based self-assessments are differentiated from the previous two by their direct observation and evaluation of a process or activity. Even though a self-assessment may provide the organization with information about its strengths and weaknesses, it does not provide a prioritization of improvement actions. Improvement actions need to be reviewed and prioritized based on the organization's mission, goals and objectives, resources, and desired level of performance.[37]

The primary elements of the self-assessment process include (a) setting recognized standards, (b) rating the standards, (c) making changes necessary to satisfy the standards, and (d) confirming achievement of the standards by external evaluators. Self-assessment provides a snapshot of how well the organization meets stated requirements, establishes methods of program delivery that meet high professional standards, and monitors the quality of its services. Standards are written statements or conditions that specify performance expectations. One of the most important (and often the most difficult) decisions to be made is the selection of indicators (or standards) for assessing HEC performance. Performance standards fall into three categories: outcome, process, or structure.[38-40]

Outcome standards. Outcome standards define desirable as well as undesirable results and can be used to benchmark performance.[41] Outcome indicators measure specific characteristics of services provided by an organization. Even though outcomes are often the typical indicators of organizational effectiveness, they can present problems in interpretation. For example, outcomes not only reflect work performance but also the application of technology as well as other characteristics of the organization's internal and external environments. Thus, cause-effect knowledge is relatively complete only when the organization can control its environment.[42] In the case of healthcare ethics outcomes, many factors beyond the HEC's locus of control (e.g., legislation, organizational polices, social norms, cultural influences, individual preferences) can have a serious impact on the services being provided and outcomes produced. According to Wolf, outcome measures associated with HEC functions (particularly ethics review/consultation) will likely be controversial due to the broad range of ethical resolutions and lack of consensus on a single best resolution.[43]

Process standards. Process standards specify how the performance capabilities of an organization are operationalized. Clearly defined processes reduce process variation, which can lead to more predictable outcomes. Even so, full compliance is not expected with process standards since a certain degree of variation may be justifiable in some situations.[44] Process measures assess the quantity or quality of organizational activities with respect to effort rather than effect or achievement. Scott contends that process measures may be more valid measures of organizational performance since they directly assess performance values.[45] But he also points out that process measures assess conformity to a given standard, not the adequacy or correctness of the standards. Wolf indicates that surveys, interviews, direct observation, and documentation review can be effectively used to evaluate HEC functions from a process perspective.[46]

Structure standards. Structure standards define the rules under which the organization is governed and services are rendered. They are the absolutes of the organization and cannot be situationally modified.[47] Structural indicators assess the capacity of the organization to perform effectively and are based on relatively stable organizational features or individual characteristics presumed to have an impact on organizational effectiveness (e.g., accreditation rating, professional staff licensure, available tools and technology, and human, physical, and financial resources). Its greatest importance is in the planning, design, and implementation of healthcare programs. Thus, structure is relevant only to the extent that it can increase or decrease the probability of good performance.[48-49] Wolf indicates that appropriate structural measures of HEC functions might include identifying the presence of (a) mechanisms for conducting ethics consultation, formulating ethics policies, and communicating information to patients and surrogates, (b) written policies, (c) library holdings on ethics subjects, (d) budget allocations and personnel to support education, and (e) ongoing ethics assessment.[50]

Donabedian suggests a certain ordering of these performance measures (structure ⇒ process ⇒ outcome) based on a fundamental functional relationship between them.[51] In essence, structure (e.g., prerequisites, organization, resources) affects process (e.g., content, configuration, rendering of services) which impacts outcomes (e.g., end product, effects of services provided).

As an evaluation strategy, self-assessment is the most desirable platform in that it is executed by those who currently are the most knowledgeable and have the highest degree of control over healthcare ethics programs—HEC chairpersons and members. Self-assessment incorporates the most beneficial elements of program evaluation (e.g., formalized structure) and internal evaluation (e.g., organizational focus) to provide a comprehensive analysis of HEC functions.

❋PRACTICAL APPLICATION

If healthcare ethics committees are to be recognized as credible components of the healthcare system, then there must be a willingness to evaluate their performance, document their success, identify opportunities for improvement, and ensure customer satisfaction. Anderson suggested that "traditional functions of ethics committees . . . could be enhanced by linking them with the healthcare organization's quality improvement program."[52] Van Allen et al. and Griener and Storch emphasized the importance of conducting a comprehensive HEC performance assessment in lieu of selectively evaluating a specific HEC function.[53,54] Due to the interdependency of HEC functions, evaluation of a single function could result in skewed data making it difficult to obtain the information necessary to plan future activities and achieve greater overall impact.

Here are some practical tips for conducting an HEC evaluation:

- *Discuss the proposed evaluation activity within the committee.* Get the support and commitment of the group and seek volunteers to champion major tasks.
- *Seek management support.* Identify the necessary organizational resources and seek additional funding (if needed).
- *Design the evaluation effort.* Clearly delineate the purpose and scope of the evaluation effort being undertaken. Will it be a comprehensive evaluation or will it be focused on a major HEC function or process? What evaluation approach (or combination of approaches) will be used? What key questions does the committee want to answer? Develop an evaluation timeline.
- *Conduct the evaluation.* Due to the volunteer nature of most healthcare ethics committees and the resultant time constraints, it is not likely that the entire committee will participate in the conduct of the evaluation. Consider identifying a small number of committee members who are interested in participating in the evaluation. Schedule time for the evaluation. It is likely that the assessment of a major function/process can take several hours. Much depends on the scope and depth of the evaluation, the selection of participants, and their knowledge of the committee's historical background and current functions. Consider scheduling separate sessions for each functional area or process being assessed.
- *Analyze the data.* The evaluation is intended to provide an opportunity for the committee to reflect on its activities and to generate topics for further discussion and consideration. Remember, if performance standards were developed, it is not necessary for the committee to perform at the level at which the standards were written. Performance standards should provide a benchmark upon which the committee's current level of development can be measured in order to plan improvement activities. Do not hesitate to seek an external interpretation of the data.
- *Report the evaluation findings to the committee.* Review and discuss evaluation findings with committee members.
- *Document the findings.* Record the evaluation participants and processes used. Maintain evaluation files for other

uses (e.g., historical, benchmarking progress, accreditation surveys).

- *Report the findings.* Decide what will be reported—major findings, data and results, alternatives, recommendations? In what format will the findings be reported—formal written report, executive summary, oral briefing with charts, newsletter/journal article, group discussion? Decide how widely evaluation findings will be distributed—who are the intended users, who else could benefit from the data being generated?

- *Take action on the findings.* Develop an action plan and timeline to address the findings. Prioritize activities. Seek volunteers to champion major tasks. Track action items and provide regular progress reports to the committee. Keep management informed on progress (as required). Seek additional resources (as required).

- *Start planning the next HEC evaluation.* That probably sounds ridiculous, but revising the process and instruments used for this evaluation while critique comments are still fresh should make the next evaluation flow smoother.

Properly planned and executed, almost any evaluation approach can be effectively used to assess healthcare ethics programs. The common elements of successful evaluation endeavors seem to be objectivity, management support, ability to change, and commitment to improvement.

Notes

1. Wolf, S. M. 1994. "Quality Assessment of Ethics in Health Care: The Accountability Revolution." *American Journal of Law & Medicine* 20(1–2): 105–28.

2. Joint Commission on Accreditation of Healthcare Organizations. 1996. *Comprehensive Accreditation Manual for Hospitals: The Official Handbook.* Oakbrook Terrace, IL: Joint Commission on Accreditation of Healthcare Organizations.

3. American Hospital Association. Technical Panel on Biomedical Ethics. *Values in Conflict: Resolving Ethical Issues in Health Care,* 2nd edition. Chicago: American Hospital Association.

4. Anderson, C. A. 1996. "Ethics Committees and Quality Improvement: A Necessary Link." *Journal of Nursing Care Quality* (October) 11(1): 22–8.

5. Callahan, D. 1992. "Ethics Committees and Social Issues: Potentials and Pitfalls." *Cambridge Quarterly of Healthcare Ethics* 1: 5–10.

6. Lewis, M. A., and C. D. Tamparo. 1993. *Medical Law, Ethics, and Bioethics in the Medical Office,* 3rd edition. Philadelphia, PA: F. A. Davis Co.

7. Thomasma, D. C. 1991. "Point and Counterpoint. Are Ethics Committees of an Enduring Nature? Yes." *HEC Forum* 3(6): 349–53.

8. Wolf, S. M. 1994. "Quality Assessment of Ethics in Health Care: The Accountability Revolution." *American Journal of Law & Medicine* 20(1–2): 105–28.

9. Shortell, S. M., and A. D. Kaluzny. 1994. *Health Care Management: Organization Design and Behavior,* 3rd edition. Albany, NY: Delmar Publishers Inc.

10. Callahan, D. 1992. "Ethics Committees and Social Issues: Potentials and Pitfalls." *Cambridge Quarterly of Healthcare Ethics* 1: 5–10.

11. Joint Commission on Accreditation of Healthcare Organizations. 1996. *Comprehensive Accreditation Manual for Hospitals: The Official Handbook.* Oakbrook Terrace, IL: Joint Commission on Accreditation of Healthcare Organizations.

12. Veney, J. E., and A. D. Kaluzny. 1991. *Evaluation and Decision Making for Health Services,* 2nd edition. Ann Arbor, MI: Health Administration Press.

13. Cranford, R. E., and A. E. Doudera. (eds.) 1994. *Institutional Ethics Committees and Health Care Decision Making.* Ann Arbor, MI: Health Administration Press.

14. Beauchamp, T. L., and J. F. Childress. 1991. *Principles of Biomedical Ethics,* 3rd edition. New York: Oxford University Press.

15. Morelli, J. E. 1990. "Should Hospital Ethic Committees Have a Budget?" *HEC Forum* 2: 203–7.

16. Ross, J. W., J. W. Glaser, D. Rasinski-Gregory, J. M. Gibson, and C. Bayley. 1993. *Health Care Ethics Committees: The Next Generation.* Chicago: American Hospital Publishing, Inc.

17. Ibid.

18. Cohen, C. B. 1992. "Avoiding 'Cloudcuckooland' in Ethics Committee Case Review: Matching Models to Issues and Concerns." *Law, Medicine & Health Care* (Winter) 20(4): 294–9.

19. Ross, J. W., J. W. Glaser, D. Rasinski-Gregory, J. M. Gibson, and C. Bayley. 1993. *Health Care Ethics Committees: The Next Generation.* Chicago: American Hospital Publishing, Inc.

20. Ibid.

21. Dobbs, R. A. 2000. Self-Assessment of Hospital Ethics Committees in New Mexico: A Study in Process Improvement, Doctoral Dissertation. Minneapolis, MN: Walden University.

22. Ross, J. W., J. W. Glaser, D. Rasinski-Gregory, J. M. Gibson, and C. Bayley. 1993. *Health Care Ethics Committees: The Next Generation.* Chicago: American Hospital Publishing, Inc.

23. Dobbs, R. A. 2000. Self-Assessment of Hospital Ethics Committees in New Mexico: A Study in Process Improvement, Doctoral Dissertation. Minneapolis, MN: Walden University.

24. Sechrest, L. and A. J. Figueredo. 1993. "Program Evaluation." *Annual Review of Psychology* 44: 645–74.

25. Franklin, J. L., and J. H. Thrasher. 1976. *An Introduction to Program Evaluation.* New York: John Wiley & Sons.

26. Ross, J. W., J. W. Glaser, D. Rasinski-Gregory, J. M. Gibson, and C. Bayley. 1993. *Health Care Ethics Committees: The Next Generation.* Chicago: American Hospital Publishing, Inc.

27. Veney, J. E., and A. D. Kaluzny. 1991. *Evaluation and Decision Making for Health Services*, 2nd edition. Ann Arbor, MI: Health Administration Press.

28. Donabedian, A. 1980. *Explorations in Quality Assessment and Monitoring: The Definition of Quality and Approaches to Its Assessment*, volume 1. Ann Arbor, MI: Health Administration Press.

29. Ibid.

30. Veney, J. E., and A. D. Kaluzny. 1991. *Evaluation and Decision Making for Health Services*, 2nd edition. Ann Arbor, MI: Health Administration Press.

31. Ibid.

32. Donabedian, A. 1980. *Explorations in Quality Assessment and Monitoring: The Definition of Quality and Approaches to Its Assessment*, volume 1. Ann Arbor, MI: Health Administration Press.

33. Love, A. J. 1991. *Internal Evaluation: Building Organizations from Within*. Newbury Park, CA: Sage Publications.

34. Wilson, P. F., and R. D. Pearson. 1995. *Performance-Based Assessments: External, Internal, and Self-Assessment Tools for Total Quality Management*. Milwaukee, WI: ASQC Quality Press.

35. Love, A. J. 1991. *Internal Evaluation: Building Organizations from Within*. Newbury Park, CA: Sage Publications.

36. Wilson, P. F., and R. D. Pearson. 1995. *Performance-Based Assessments: External, Internal, and Self-Assessment Tools for Total Quality Management*. Milwaukee, WI: ASQC Quality Press.

37. Saco, R. M. 1997. "The Criteria: A Looking Glass to American's Understanding of Quality." *Quality Progress* 30(11): 89–96.

38. Donabedian, A. 1980. *Explorations in Quality Assessment and Monitoring: The Definition of Quality and Approaches to Its Assessment*, volume 1. Ann Arbor, MI: Health Administration Press.

39. Love, A. J. 1991. *Internal Evaluation: Building Organizations from Within*. Newbury Park, CA: Sage Publications.

40. Scott, W. R. 1981. *Organizations: Rational, Natural, and Open Systems*. Englewood Cliffs, NJ: Prentice-Hall, Inc.

41. Katz, J. M., and E. Green. 1997. *Managing Quality: A Guide to System-Wide Performance Management in Health Care*, 2nd edition. St. Louis, MO: Mosby-Year Book, Inc.

42. Scott, W. R. 1981. *Organizations: Rational, Natural, and Open Systems*. Englewood Cliffs, NJ: Prentice-Hall, Inc.

43. Wolf, S. M. 1994. "Quality Assessment of Ethics in Health Care: The Accountability Revolution." *American Journal of Law & Medicine* 20(1–2): 105–28.

44. Katz, J. M., and E. Green. 1997. *Managing Quality: A Guide to System-Wide Performance Management in Health Care*, 2nd edition. St. Louis, MO: Mosby-Year Book, Inc.

45. Scott, W. R. 1981. *Organizations: Rational, Natural, and Open Systems*. Englewood Cliffs, NJ: Prentice-Hall, Inc.

46. Wolf, S. M. 1994. "Quality Assessment of Ethics in Health Care: The

Accountability Revolution." *American Journal of Law & Medicine* 20(1–2): 105–28.

47. Katz, J. M., and E. Green. 1997. *Managing Quality: A Guide to System-Wide Performance Management in Health Care*, 2nd edition. St. Louis, MO: Mosby-Year Book, Inc.

48. Donabedian, A. 1980. *Explorations in Quality Assessment and Monitoring: The Definition of Quality and Approaches to Its Assessment*, volume 1. Ann Arbor, MI: Health Administration Press.

49. Scott, W. R. 1981. *Organizations: Rational, Natural, and Open Systems.* Englewood Cliffs, NJ: Prentice-Hall, Inc.

50. Wolf, S. M. 1994. "Quality Assessment of Ethics in Health Care: The Accountability Revolution." *American Journal of Law & Medicine* 20(1–2): 105–28.

51. Donabedian, A. 1980. *Explorations in Quality Assessment and Monitoring: The Definition of Quality and Approaches to Its Assessment*, volume 1. Ann Arbor, MI: Health Administration Press. 83.

52. Anderson, C. A. 1996. "Ethics Committees and Quality Improvement: A Necessary Link." *Journal of Nursing Care Quality* (October) 11(1): 27.

53. Van Allen, E., D. G. Moldow, and R. Cranford. 1989. "Evaluating Ethics Committees." *Hastings Center Report* (Sept/Oct) 19(5): 23–4.

54. Griener, G. G., and J. L. Storch. 1992. "Hospital Ethics Committees: Problems in Evaluation." *HEC Forum* 4(1): 5–18.

GENDER DISCRIMINATION:
ROLLING MEADOWS COMMUNITY HOSPITAL

ROLLING MEADOWS Community Hospital is a 200-bed acute care facility located in an affluent suburb of a major metropolitan area in the Midwest. The hospital is highly regarded within the community, especially for its obstetrics program with its innovative birthing center, its ambulatory care program, and its geriatrics center. The hospital is supported by a large group practice of young, well-trained primary care physicians who occupy an adjacent medical office building owned by the hospital. Amidst the last decade of turmoil in healthcare delivery, Rolling Meadows has remained financially strong. Indeed, it has prospered in an environment that quickly became dominated by managed care in recent years.

Rolling Meadows was well positioned for such changes. Its financial stability, its strong primary care base, and its modern facilities predicted success. In addition, located among the rolling meadows for which it is named, adjacent to an exclusive golf course, makes it a desirable place of employment for professional and nonprofessional staff alike.

John Waverly has been the CEO of Rolling Meadows for five years. The governing board for Rolling Meadows conducted a national search five years ago and rigorously recruited the 42-year-old John who was then an up and coming HMO executive on the West Coast. The board continues to congratulate itself on its foresight and wisdom. John was just what Rolling Meadows needed to make the hospital a major player in the then emerging managed care market. The hospital has thrived under John's leadership and he has been well compensated for his efforts. In addition, John continues to enjoy the favor of a governing board, which although conservative, has remained supportive of John's innovative management style. John is the envy of his peers in other more beleaguered healthcare institutions and, at age 47, he feels good about his professional achievements and status.

In retrospect, his decision to take the CEO position at Rolling Meadows had been a good one. At the time of his recruitment, John had major reservations about relocating to the Midwest, especially to the conservative community surrounding Rolling Meadows. He wasn't sure his wife and children would easily adjust. And indeed, they have never fully embraced this community, a fact which continues to be a source of tension in John's life.

In the beginning, John had also been uneasy about his credentials and how well his educational background would translate to the delivery side of healthcare. John knew he would have to work especially hard to compensate for his lack of hospital experience.

Six months ago, John hired a bright, ambitious postgraduate fellow from a prestigious university program in hospital administration. At the time, John was about to enter into discussions with two nearby powerful healthcare financing and delivery systems, both of which had expressed interest in Rolling Meadows becoming a part of their multi-hospital structure. John knew that these discussions and evaluations of any proposals emanating from them would be time consuming and demand a great deal of research and preparation. Having a capable postgraduate fellow on board to perform staff work appeared to be a win/win situation. It would provide valuable experience for the fellow as well as needed manpower for the organization. Also, John especially liked the idea of working with someone well schooled in the latest academic trends in healthcare administration.

Over the past six months, the partnership proved to be as fruitful as promised. The CEO and his young protégé worked closely together. Long hours and weekends were required and Rolling Meadows benefited greatly from their hard work. John and his young protégé found themselves celebrating success after success. It was a most enjoyable partnership. She admired and respected John. He was flattered by her admiration. He found himself seeking out opportunities to spend more and more time with her. She began accompanying him to all of his meetings even those unrelated to her assigned projects. He looked for educational conferences in attractive locations where the two of them enjoyed fine dining and upscale accommodations.

Now, her fellowship was nearing its close and she approached John about her future career plans. Her performance evaluations had been outstanding, as indeed had been her accomplishments. Rolling Meadows had profited greatly from her efforts, and she fully anticipated to be rewarded with a post-fellowship position. After all, many of her peers already had experienced job offers from their fellowship organizations and they had no significant accomplishments to report from their fellowship experiences. John had been an outstanding mentor and her admiration and respect for him bordered on "hero worship."

John was not unprepared for this discussion. After much thought, he had decided it would not be prudent for him to offer her a position at Rolling Meadows. He candidly explained the situation to her. Her performance was outstanding, her professionalism had been noted by many, and she was a brilliant strategist. But, he said, he was personally attracted to her and he felt this attraction was reciprocated and he believed that if they continued to spend time together this attraction would escalate to a physical relationship.

He offered to help her in her job search by providing impeccable references and contacting his colleagues in progressive, innovative organizations where her talents would be showcased. She was astonished and humiliated. With her accomplishments and her close relationship with John, she assumed a position for her would be readily available. She felt used and betrayed. Angry, she said this constituted nothing more than sexual harassment. John believed this to be an idle threat and that reason would overcome her emotional outburst.

The following day, John received a phone call from a member of the governing board informing him that an executive session of the board had been scheduled to discuss this "appalling situation" and what action should be taken to avert a lawsuit. He told John to be prepared to respond to the allegations at this meeting and if they were accurate, he should consider resignation to spare the hospital any adverse publicity.

John was surprised by the call and by the tone of the conversation but he felt confident that he had done nothing wrong. In fact, he believed he had honestly appraised the potential dangers of his relationship with the fellow and had avoided any misconduct. He believed his actions had been in the best interests of the organization and that the governing board would agree.

ETHICS ISSUES

Adherence to Hospital's Ethical Standards and Values Are John's actions in this situation consistent with the hospital's ethical standards and values?

Adherence to Professional Codes of Ethics Is John's conduct in this situation consistent with the professional codes of ethics as promulgated by the professional organizations representing healthcare executives and hospitals?

Legal Implications Do John's actions in this situation constitute sexual harassment? If so, are John and the hospital both liable for these actions? Or could this situation be viewed as a case of gender discrimination?

Leadership Responsibilities Was John's conduct in this situation consistent with the role and responsibility that is inherent to the position of CEO of a healthcare organization?

Expectations of a Mentorship Program What is the role and responsibilities of a mentor? Of a protégé? Upon completion of a postgraduate fellowship, what can each of the participants expect to have achieved? In this case has the postgraduate fellowship met or failed its expectations?

Organizational Implications Has this situation and specifically John's actions had any impact on other employees within the organization? Has the "image" of the organization been affected by this situation? Are there financial implications to John's actions?

Justice and Fairness Has the postgraduate fellow in this case been treated fairly? Is John being treated fairly by the governing board considering his candor and honesty regarding this situation?

DISCUSSION

A Question of Wrongdoing/Legal Implications

The fundamental issue in this case may well be did John, in fact, do anything wrong?

It appears that formal allegations of sexual harassment may be forthcoming. Do John's actions here constitute sexual harassment? John would vehemently deny any explicit or implicit actions or expressions that would suggest sexual harassment. He admits to his attraction to the fellow but insists that the long hours worked together, the meetings, and out-of-town conferences were work related and she was in no way coerced to spend this time with him. Indeed, he would argue that she seemed to be attracted to him and if anything, she seemed to encourage his attentions with frequent flattery and expressions of gratitude for the time and effort he was putting into her fellowship experience.

There are those who would argue that John's superior position as CEO and her subordinate position as postgraduate fellow constitutes a power advantage for John that "implies" coercion, whether or not overt coercion exists. But, if John and his protégé both willingly and actively participated in this relationship, does that not imply acceptable activity between two consenting adults? And as such, would not this relationship be consistent with prevailing societal norms, and therefore lacking coercion?

If not sexual harassment, then perhaps John is guilty of sexual misconduct. There was, however, no sexual or physical behavior on the part of John or the fellow. In fact, there was no expression of desire or intimacy involved. To himself, John would admit flirtation, but nothing more. Is attraction, unacted upon, a form of sexual misconduct? "Adultery of the heart," so to speak, as admitted by one recent past president? There are common religious beliefs that delineate clearly between desire or intention and action. These beliefs suggest that it is the action that is "sinful" and if the "evil" desires are overcome by will and hence not acted upon, such behavior may be considered virtuous. In this case, John chose not to take the relationship to the next level. That is, assuming that the choice was his alone to make.

Or do we have a case of gender discrimination here? Would this postgraduate fellow have been offered a position with the organization if she had been a male? Of course, there are no guarantees that each high-performing postgraduate fellow *will* be offered a position upon completion of the fellowship, but it can be argued that it is a somewhat common practice among healthcare organizations.

Were there financial improprieties here? Were the out-of-state conferences necessary or were they merely boondoggles? Is it wrong to consider these conferences in upscale locations as a well-deserved and appropriate reward for high-performing staff who may be putting in long hours in lowly compensated positions especially if they are infrequent and have educational merit?

Is John's conduct in this case simply an example of bad judgment? Were John's actions in this situation motivated by a sense of power and a belief that his status and accomplishments placed him above the need to avoid any appearances of improprieties? John will argue that his actions were always in the best interests of the organization. He is able to cite significant accomplishments as a result of this mentor-protégé relationship. According to John, his intentions were always to serve as a diligent preceptor and he believes the fellowship has been an educationally rewarding experience for the fellow. He is stunned that anyone on the governing board would consider his actions to be anything *other* than in the best interests of the organization. After all, it was for the good of the organization that he had denied a position to this fellow. John believes the only thing he may be guilty of is misplaced honesty and he greatly regrets the admission of his attraction to the postgraduate fellow.

In its upcoming review of this case, it would appear that the governing board members must, as much as is possible, set aside their personal standards of conduct and rely on the hospital's standards and policies and professional codes of ethics if they are to make a fair and just assessment of this situation.

Adherence to Hospital's Ethical Standards and Values

In resolving the issues of this case, it would certainly be advantageous to have the ability to refer to the hospitals' ethical standards and values. Indeed, assistance in the resolution of ethical questions is ample justification for written standards of ethical practice within an organization. Such written standards also provide valuable guidelines for the day-to-day professional and business operations of an organization.

The American Hospital Association Management Advisory on Ethical Conduct for Health Care Institutions makes it clear that the governing board has the responsibility for establishing the ethical standards that guide the organization's operations.[1] Legal and accreditation requirements address this obligation as well.

Emanating from the hospital's mission statement, these ethical standards frequently reflect the mission of the organization in responding to the needs of its community and reflecting the prevailing standards of behavior within its community. In this particular case, while no such written standards of ethical conduct or value statement are in place, the mission statement for Rolling Meadows does reference "family values" regarding its commitment to serve its community through state-of-the-art programs in family practice, obstetrics, and gynecology and geriatrics. The service area for Rolling Meadows is family oriented, religious, and conservative and the board members representing this community reflect these same values. Under these circumstances, is it safe to assume that John's behavior will be judged within the same framework as his colleagues in other healthcare organizations? If not, is this fair?

Adherence to Professional Codes of Ethics

The *Code of Ethics* of the American College of Healthcare Executives provides guidelines for ethical conduct for healthcare executives. It identifies standards of ethical behavior for healthcare executives in their professional relationships and in their personal relationships especially when their "conduct directly relates to the role and identity of the healthcare executive." The *Code* advises that healthcare executives should serve as "moral advocates" and should "act in ways that will merit the trust, confidence and respect" of all. In doing so "healthcare executives should lead lives that embody an exemplary system of values and ethics."[2] If these standards are to be applied to this case, the key word here may be "exemplary."

In its section on Responsibilities to Employees the *Code* obligates healthcare executives to "work to ensure a working environment that is free from harassment, sexual and other; coercion of any kind . . . and discrimination on the basis of race, creed, color, sex, ethnic origin, age or disability."[3]

In addition to this professional *Code of Ethics*, the board may wish to reference the American Hospital Associations Management Advisory on Ethical Conduct for Health Care Institutions. This advisory notes that healthcare organizations have an obligation to "conduct themselves in an ethical manner that emphasizes a basic community service orientation and justifies the public trust."[4] This directive may or may not apply in this case.

Organizational Implications

Has this situation and specifically John's behavior had any impact on other employees within the organization? Typically, regardless of how discreet the individuals within any "special" relationship may be, it is quickly perceived as such by the majority of the workforce who are in contact with the participants. This is especially true when the very visible CEO position is involved. Such "special" relationships are often a frequent topic of office gossip and speculation and are bound to be an unneeded distraction at best and a threat to the credibility of management at worst. Regardless of what the participants may choose to believe, such things as favoritism, physical attractions, and flirtations are always obvious to the outside observers and do have some impact on the functioning of the organization, albeit negligible in some cases. If these office rumors filter outside of the organization into other more public domains, as they often do, the image of the organization and the effectiveness of the CEO may suffer.

In a recent poll conducted by the Society for Human Resource Management, 75 percent of United States companies surveyed discourage or prohibit workplace romances and cite the potential for retaliation if a romance ends as their rationale. Twenty-seven percent of United States companies have written or widely understood policies about dating among coworkers, and although 55 percent of companies permit workplace romances, they do discourage them.[5]

Finally, are there financial improprieties evident in John's actions here? The answer to this question must follow a careful review of the hospital's policies related to educational conferences and business travel. Adherence to these policies must be uniform among the staff, including the CEO.

Leadership and Power

"The essence of leadership is elusive," states Austin Ross in his book, *Cornerstones of Leadership for Healthcare Executives.*[6] All of the experts will agree however that leaders have certain common characteristics. Often cited characteristics include vision, integrity, intelligence, initiative, interpersonal skills, ethics, and flexibility, to name a few. There are also some agreed upon expectations of leaders. They are expected to serve as positive role models, to motivate staff and employees, to be committed to the organization's mission and goals, to be responsive to the needs of the community, to establish ethical standards, and to be of strong moral character.

Indeed, John Griffith reminds us that the higher the rank of the leader, the more important his or her moral character is. In fact, he says that "top management and governance must be visibly moral."[7] Austin Ross says leaders are "guardians of ethical conduct" and a leader's questionable conduct "leads to declining staff confidence in ethics and values" and an "erosion of self respect among the organization's workforce."[8] Ross cautions leaders to avoid preferential treatment of staff. There is a tendency among executives, he says, to liberally reward their immediate subordinates for jobs well done when others in the organization may perform equally well, yet go unrewarded. While this behavior may reflect a need to "purchase personal loyalty," it is often viewed as unfair.[9]

We have all heard the expression; "It's lonely at the top." Perhaps we have even said it on occasion. Unfortunately, to be effective, a leader must willingly take on this hardship. "Just as the captain of a ship enjoys a solitary voyage, leaders must be able to tolerate loneliness."[10] Too often, the job is just not that much fun. The leader may enjoy friendship and confidences among professional colleagues in other organizations (albeit noncompetitors), but not within one's organization without the risk of compromising the leader's position.

Further complicating the role and responsibilities of leaders is the issue of professional power. John Worthley defines professional power as the "ability to influence or affect the life of another by virtue of the professional position one holds."

In his book, *The Ethics of the Ordinary in Healthcare*, Worthley provides a primer on the sources of professional power. They are as follows: 1) coercive power—subordinates treat superiors with deference and compliance out of fear of reprisal, 2) connective power—the one in power is needed for access so he/she is given power and compliance with his/her whims in order to gain favor or avoid disfavor, 3) presumed expertise—the one in power is perceived to have expertise or knowledge that is needed so deference is paid, 4) information—the one in power has information or access to information that is needed so deference is paid, 5) rewards—it is believed that the one in power will bestow rewards if deference is paid, and 6) legitimacy—the one in authority is granted power by virtue of his/her position.[11]

Experienced healthcare professionals may have observed yet another dynamic which for lack of an official label could be termed paternalistic power. The subordinates in this scenario seek the approval of the "parent" authority and want nothing more than to please the superior. Taken to extremes, the subordinate may begin to adopt manners of dress, appearances, and work habits of the superior. If the behavior borders on the obsequious, the subordinate may be ridiculed by other employees and called a "yes man" or worse. Most subordinates with this behavior are seeking career advancement. There are some subordinates, however, who want nothing more than to please the boss and be liked by him or her. No doubt, there are ample psychologists who would be more than willing to trace such behavior to an unfulfilled child-parent relationship.

The behavior of the superior in this dynamic can be interesting, as well. While some superiors may feel flattered and enjoy such subordinate behavior, others may dismiss it and seek more original thinking and intellectual challenge on the part of subordinates. As in all circumstances, the leader does, in fact, take the lead in defining the patterns of behavior that are to prevail within an organization.

An additional source of power for executives, whether in healthcare or in the corporate world, is the rituals and symbols that define the "executive office" and imbue power to those who inhabit it. Berger and Luckmann posit the theory that all reality is socially constructed by the interactions of the participants. They believe that symbols and rituals structure and influence this interaction and distribute power accordingly. The corner office, the executive furniture, the Mont Blanc pens, the executive attire, the framed diploma all signify authority and set apart the executives from the less powerful employees.[12]

Worthley notes that professionals often underestimate the level of power that they exercise. In fact, he warns that it can be dangerous when the powerful are unaware of the power they wield.[13] It can be equally dangerous, however, when the powerful become so aware and so seduced by power that the powerful acts in arrogant disregard of the norms, laws, and standards intended for all within a profession, an organization, or a society. The idea of hubris, excessive pride or self-inflation, and its downfall is often noted in mythology and in history. In Greek mythology, the hero aspiring to be like the gods was usually punished by death.[14] In modern times, political figures abound who believed they were above the law and suffered a demolished career and reputation as a result. Less conspicuous but more common in healthcare management is the highly regarded, committed leader who may develop a sense of entitlement regarding the "perks" of the position as a result of the long hours and personal sacrifices that he or she has endured.

Finally, there are those leaders struggling with a desire to do the right thing who are confronted with ethical dilemmas and ambiguities. The close scrutiny of their actions enjoyed by most senior-level executives makes them especially vulnerable to question.

Griffith reminds us that "it is not necessary to be perfect to be a moral leader."[15] Indeed, the American Heart Association Committee on Ethics noted that: "ethical practice in the profession may well stem more from sensitive awareness of one's self and how one is actually impacting on persons and situation than from any specific knowledge."[16] Griffith tells us that leaders "promote moral virtue by example" and that "strong leadership can promote morality among subordinates" whereas weak leadership fosters lax morality. Moral leadership begins at the top because those at the top have the "greatest freedom to act."[17]

Austin Ross advises those in leadership positions to take advantage of the many resources available for ethical guidance including professional organizations, university programs, publications, ethical consultants, networking, and the Internet. Ross reminds leaders that their best source of guidance remains the organization's mission statement, which should help to define the ethical standards of the organization and provide a sense of purpose and direction to staff.[18]

Sex Discrimination and Sexual Harassment

Sex discrimination is against the law and has been since Congress passed the Civil Rights Act of 1964. This law, along with various state and local statutes, prohibits discrimination based on race, sex, religion, age, national origin, and disability. Title VII of the Civil Rights Act of 1964 prohibits discrimination in private employment with respect to compensation for and the terms, conditions and privileges of employment. This includes hiring, firing, promotion, transfer, job training, and apprenticeship decisions. The Civil Rights Act of 1991 awarded to victims of such discrimination the right to jury trials and compensatory and punitive damages. The Equal Employment Opportunity Commission (EEOC) is the federal agency established to administer the law.[19]

Sex discrimination was not part of the Civil Rights Act of 1964 as it was originally written. It was attached at the last minute by conservative southern opponents of the bill who thought that something as "ludicrous" as equality of the sexes would surely cause the bill to founder. The bill passed and became law but the EEOC took no action against sex discrimination in employment for several years until pressure from the women's movement made it an issue. A case was subsequently made that sexual harassment is in fact a form of sex discrimination. In 1980, the EEOC defined sexual harassment as a form of sex discrimination prohibited by the Civil Rights Act and, in 1986, the U.S. Supreme Court held that sexual harassment on the job was a form of sex discrimination.[20]

In the case of Rolling Meadows Community Hospital, an examination of the possibility of disparate treatment because of gender may be in order. If an employee was treated less favorably because of gender or was treated differently *and* less favorably, it may be a case of disparate treatment and discrimination. The "victim" must show that the employer intended to discriminate because of gender. This means that the complainant must show that he/she applied and was qualified for a job or promotion that the employer was seeking to fill; that the employee was denied; and that the employer continued to seek applications. The employer does not need to prove a lack of discrimination. Employers are given a great deal of latitude in this area and can disguise questionable employment practices as business decisions. The complainant, on the other hand, must show direct evidence such as derogatory statements by the employer *or* comparative evidence such as similar situations where others were treated more favorably, or that the employer acted contrary to its own policies.[21]

While sexual harassment is a form of sex discrimination, it is not always as easy to define. Typically, the legal issues will focus on whether the conduct in question is sexual in nature, unreasonable, severe, and unwelcome.[22] Title VII of the Civil Rights Act speaks to sexual harassment as unwelcome sexual conduct of two types: 1) quid pro quo or sexual favors for job benefits; and 2) hostile work environment where the employee is forced to endure unpleasant conduct because of gender. In quid pro quo situations, the harasser must be one who has authority over the victim's job and benefits. In hostile work environment, any conduct of a sexual nature that interferes with an employee's work is considered "hostile."[23]

Most experts agree that a key determinant of sexual harassment is whether the conduct is unwelcome. But this is not always readily apparent. The EEOC has stated that "because sexual attraction may often play a role in the day-to-day social exchange between employees, the distinction between invited, uninvited but welcome, offensive but tolerated, and flatly rejected advances may well be difficult to discover."[24]

Office romances are an inevitable fact of life. According to a 1994 American Management Association survey, 80 percent of those surveyed have had or know of an office romance. Some cited reasons include more women in the workforce and an increasing time spent at work.[25] A 1997 survey by the Society for Human Resources Management found that 70 percent of companies that had policies on workplace romances banned romance between supervisors and subordinates. The human resources managers also reported that 55 percent of those involved in office romances got married, 28 percent of these resulted in complaints of favoritism by coworkers, and 24 percent led to decreased productivity among those involved.[26]

It is generally agreed that the most "dangerous liaisons" occur between superiors and subordinates. The supervisor undermines his/her authority, jeopardizes his/her working relationships with other reports and is often accused of favoritism. In fact, the subordinate may be treated less favorably in an attempt to cover up the relationship. Sometimes the subordinate involved in the relationship is viewed as an informant and isolated by coworkers.[27] Charges of sexual harassment against one in authority are often scrutinized more closely than others because of the strong possibility of abuse of power. In fact, very little conduct of a sexual nature is needed in a supervisor-subordinate relationship to warrant such an investigation.[28] Thus, some employers have strict policies prohibiting supervisors from dating subordinates.[29]

According to Alex Fryer and Carol Ostrom, "Like Clinton, most CEOs can survive office affairs." They report that in their research, CEOs are rarely fired for sexual misconduct. Governing boards appear to be more interested in financial performances than in their CEO's sexual escapades.[30] But sexual misconduct, and especially charges of sexual harassment, can be extremely costly to business and employers are almost automatically responsible for the actions of a superior when a subordinate makes such charges.[31] The *average* cost to defend against a sexual harassment claim is $100,000 and the *average* settlement is $15,000.[32] In 1998, Mitsubishi Motor Manufacturing of America settled what was probably the most globally publicized claim of sexual harassment ever for $34 million.

The less tangible, but perhaps even more damaging effects of sexual harassment claims are distrust of management, high turnover, tarnished employer image, loss of productivity, poor product quality, and customer and shareholder dissatisfaction.[33]

Insuring the company against employee sexual harassment litigation is hardly inexpensive. Policy premiums typically cost about $10,000 for each $1 million coverage. Insurance usually covers legal costs, back pay, and compensatory damages but not punitive awards.[34]

There are some who argue that the costs of sexual harassment claims hurt more than just the individual companies involved. Elizabeth Larson argues that the laws have stimulated the growth of a new industry of consultants that may, in fact, foster complaints. Increased complaints mean more litigation, decreased productivity, absenteeism, employer turnover, and low morale. In fact, she contends that " . . . teaching . . . women to look for harassment and slights . . . in the workplace hurts everyone in the long run—most of all women."[35]

Others say the proliferation of sexual harassment claims in the last decade is simply a result of the government overregulating the workplace and that most of the claims are false and a costly waste of time.[36] Such critics suggest that false claims may be filed because the complainant despises the boss, was rejected by a superior, was humiliated or made to feel inferior, hates the company, or is just seeking financial gain.[37]

Regardless, sexual harassment *is* against the law and the employer is responsible for establishing strong policies prohibiting sexual harassment in the workplace, effective investigative procedures, and comprehensive training programs for all employees, management, and governing board members.[38]

Sexual harassment is not a simple issue and its complexities make it a major ethical challenge for organizations. Smart organizations will meet this challenge and commit the necessary resources to create a working environment free from harassment because they know it is costly not to do so.

Mentoring

Numerous research studies have indicated that having a mentor significantly affects one's professional development and career advancement. According to a 1986 Korn/Ferry International Study, corporate leaders rated mentoring second only to education as a significant factor in their success. Two recent Catalyst studies, *On the Line: Women's Career Advancement* and *Women in Engineering: An Untapped Resource* substantiate that the mentoring that women receive from influential colleagues is critical to their career success.[39] Michael Zey interviewed 150 executives from Fortune 500 corporations and noted that mentoring was frequently cited as the single most important factor contributing to one's corporate success.[40]

A postgraduate fellowship is "a structured, preceptor-directed, planned program of development that consists of a learning and working clinical experience in a healthcare facility . . . after the conferring of the academic degree."[41] A fellowship provides an opportunity for the protégé or fellow to gain real-world experience in his/her professional field, to refine skills, and to test academic concepts.[42]

The preceptor or mentor is typically a senior-level executive who is interested in teaching and sharing experiences, insights, and knowledge with young professionals about to embark upon their careers. Some view mentoring as a mechanism whereby executives can contribute to their professional field and assist in the professional preparation of future colleagues.

The mentor must be an "emotionally secure" individual with high ethical standards and values who behaves in a rational, consistent manner. This is important because the mentor is serving as a role model and teaching by example. The protégé will often adopt the demeanor and value system of the mentor and will typically retain this learned work philosophy throughout his/her career.[43]

The mentor, because of position and experience, can provide the direction and guidance that the protégé needs to achieve career goals. The mentor serves as a teacher and protector, providing learning opportunities. The mentor allows the protégé to make mistakes but intervenes when circumstances become too difficult or complex.[44] To achieve these goals, the mentor must be professionally competent, enjoy a favorable professional reputation and network of colleagues, and be willing to commit the required time to be an effective mentor.[45] Time is a precious commodity in the life of an executive and mentoring takes time. Minimally, the mentor must plan the fellowship experience, assign meaningful projects, confer at least weekly with the protégé to assess progress, and provide honest evaluation. Most importantly, the protégé must have access to the mentor.

It is this "access to the boss" that sometimes creates problems among other employees who may feel that the protégé enjoys special privilege. The perception of favoritism is just one of the pitfalls of mentoring. Austin Ross warns those who mentor to avoid falling prey to an "over developed personal ego" where they only teach what they believe to be true. He also warns of the dangers of "mutual dependency" as a result of the close relationship shared by mentors and protégés.[46] Working so closely with each other, sharing thoughts and spending great amounts of time together can also serve to predispose the principal participants in a fellowship to a romantic relationship. This possibility could help to explain in some measure why some men are reluctant to mentor women.

Given the fact that most CEOs are men, gender could potentially serve as a barrier to desirable mentorship situations for women. Research has shown that women face certain other barriers to developing worthwhile mentorship relationships as well. A 1990 Department of Education study found that women face several obstacles to being accepted by a male mentor. These include: lack of access to information networks; tokenism; stereotypes; socialization practices; norms regarding cross-gender relationships; and women's reliance on ineffective power bases.[47]

Indeed, the American College of Healthcare Executives study, *A Comparison of the Career Attainments of Men and Women Healthcare Executives,* found that when asked about critical factors to promotions, job performance was most often mentioned by men while women also mentioned having a mentor, opportunities for visibility with senior management, being willing to work long hours, resembling senior managers in appearance or style, and having informal social contacts with senior managers away from work.[48] In addition, when asked if they were not hired, promoted, or had not received fair compensation because of their gender, significant differences were reported. Twelve percent of women compared to 4 percent of men said they were not hired because of their gender; 33 percent of women compared to 4 percent of men said they were not promoted because of gender; and 48 percent of women compared to none of the men said they did not receive fair compensation because of gender.[49] And finally, the majority of women surveyed felt that more men possess beneficial mentor-protégé relationships than they do.[50]

One explanation offered for this belief is that male managers have more access to informal executive networks than female managers and that these informal networks tend to be the "dominant organizational coalitions" that provide better access to mentors. The prevalence of this dynamic makes it especially important for women to have interaction with senior-level executives through fellowships, membership in professional societies like the American College of Healthcare Executives, service on local or statewide healthcare committees, and the like. The absence of such executive interaction has been found to significantly impede the career advancement of women.[51]

Having executive interaction and mentorship that crosses gender lines does provide potential for inappropriate sexual behavior on the part of one or both of the participants. Recognizing this, the American Medical Association has published guidelines for preventing sexual harassment that include a code of behavior for teacher-learner relationships. This code notes that the "teacher-learner relationship should be based on mutual trust, respect and responsibility . . . carried out in a professional manner, in a learning environment that places strong focus on education, high quality patient care and ethical conduct." The teacher is expected to provide instruction, guidance, inspiration, and leadership. The learner is expected to commit the effort to acquire the necessary knowledge and skill to become an effective physician. In addition to defining and prohibiting sexual harassment, this code of behavior specifically addresses consensual amorous relationships between teacher and student noting that the fundamental power imbalance between the two partners and the possibility of biased evaluations, either positively or negatively, make these relationships unethical. Because of the "inherent inequality in status and power," . . . "the potential for sexual exploitation exists despite the voluntary nature of the relationship."[52]

Notes

1. *Ethical Conduct for Healthcare Institutions.* 1992. Chicago: American Hospital Association, Introduction.
2. *Code of Ethics.* 2000. Chicago: American College of Healthcare Executives, Preamble.
3. *Code of Ethics.* 2000. Chicago: American College of Healthcare Executives, Section II, C, 3.
4. *Ethical Conduct for Healthcare Institutions.* 1992. Chicago: American Hospital Association, Introduction.
5. MacIntyre, J. 2000. "Facts of Life." *Spirit,* June, 2000, 46.

6. Ross, A., *Cornerstones of Leadership for Healthcare Executives*. Ann Arbor, MI: Health Administration Press. 1.

7. Griffith, J. R. 1996. *The Moral Challenges of Health Care Management*. Chicago, IL: Health Administration Press. 137.

8. Ross, 26.

9. Ross, 26.

10. Ross, 38.

11. Worthley, J. A. 1997. *The Ethics of the Ordinary in Healthcare*. Chicago: Health Administration Press. 62–4.

12. Berger, P. L., and T. Luckmann. 1967. *The Social Construction of Reality*. Borden City, New York: Anchor Books, Doubleday and Co. 91.

13. Worthley, 63

14. O'Neil, J. R. 1994. *The Paradox of Success*. New York: G. P. Putnam's Sons. 86.

15. Griffith, 136.

16. American Heart Association Committee on Ethics. 1980. "A Perspective on Teaching Medical Ethics." 6.

17. Griffith, 136.

18. Ross, 28.

19. Outten, W. N., R. J. Rabin, and L.R. Lepman, *The Basic ACLU Guide to the Rights of Employees and Union Members*. Carbondale, IL: Southern Illinois University Press. 149–53.

20. Petrocelli, W. and B. K. Repa. 1998. *Sexual Harassment on the Job*. Berkeley, CA: Nolo Press. 1/19–21.

21. Outten, 149–53.

22. Petrocelli, 2/2.

23. Outten, 213–4.

24. Outten, 215.

25. McUsic, T. 1999. "Office Romances Pick Up Steam, Author Says." *Albuquerque Journal* November 15, I1.

26. Glover, C. 1998. "President's Affair Could Impact Business Policies on Romance." *Albuquerque Journal*, August 30, A14.

27. Neville, K. 2000. *Internal Affairs*. New York: McGraw Hill. 109.

28. Petrocelli, 2/5.

29. Petrocelli, 3/12.

30. Fryer A. and C. Ostrom. 1998. "Like Clinton, Most CEOs Can Survive Office Affairs." *Albuquerque Journal*, November 29, H1.

31. Petrocelli, 2/5.

32. Neville, 60.

33. Neville, 206.

34. Neville, 202.

35. Gerdes, L. I. 1999. *Sexual Harassment: Current Controversies*. San Diego, CA: Greenhaven Press, Inc. 53–60.

36. Neville, 19.

37. Neville, 86–7.

38. Neville, 219

39. Neville, 223.

40. Ross, 70.

41. Foundation of the American College of Healthcare Executives. 1996. Research Series No. 5, *A Comparison of the Career Attainments of Men and Women Healthcare Executives*. Chicago, IL. 9.

42. Duran, B. and C. Hall. 1997. *Handbook Public Health Practicum*. Albuquerque, NM: University of New Mexico. 1.

43. Ross, 72, 73.

44. Neville, 223.

45. Duran, 6–7.

46. Ross, 77.

47. Catalyst, "Working with Business to Effect Change for Women." 1993. Report based on a study by catalyst for the Glass Ceiling Commission of the U.S. Department of Labor.

48. Foundation of the American College of Healthcare Executives Research Series, No. 5, 13.

49. Foundation of the American College of Healthcare Executives Research Series, No. 5, 14.

50. Foundation of the American College of Healthcare Executives Research Series, No. 5, 17.

51. Walsh, A. and S. Barkowiski. 1995. "Gender Differences in Factors Affecting Health Care Administration Career Development." *Hospital and Health Services Administration* 40(4): 265–75.

52. American Medical Association. 1990. *Guidelines for Establishing Sexual Harassment Prevention and Grievance Procedures and Statement on Teacher-Learner Relationships in Medical Education Code of Behavior*. 7–11.

PHYSICIAN IMPAIRMENT:
UNIVERSITY HOSPITAL

U NIVERSITY HOSPITAL had long been designated as the Level I Trauma Center serving a tri-county area of a northwestern state. It enjoys a favorable reputation among healthcare professionals and the public it serves. Its teaching, research, and patient care programs are of the highest caliber. Its trauma center is nationally known for its excellent medical staff and the resident physicians who train there are in demand all across the country upon graduation from the program.

Jan Adams has been the second-shift supervisor for the OR for ten years. She knows her job and is well liked and highly respected by staff and physicians alike. She makes certain that the surgeons follow protocol and never "get out of hand." And she probably knows more about the skill levels of the surgical staff than the majority of the surgeons themselves.

Jan likes working second shift and she likes working with trauma patients. There is a great deal of gratification in the life-saving immediacy so visible with trauma patients. Friday nights have always been the busiest night of the week for trauma and this Friday was no exception. The helicopter was on its way in with a 42-year-old victim of an automobile accident who had been struck head on by a high-speeding drunk driver going the wrong way on the interstate.

The resident, Dr. Truman, was already scrubbing as were the two other house staff who would be assisting. The scrub nurse and circulating nurse had the room set up and were waiting. Dr. Spalding, the trauma surgeon on call, was on his way to the hospital and the anesthesiologist was setting up when the patient arrived. Things looked grim, lots of bleeding, vitals fading. Dr. Truman quickly prepped and draped the unconscious patient and readied to make his incision. Dr. Spalding had still not arrived but Dr. Truman knew he had to proceed if the patient was going to make it.

Jan was concerned that Dr. Spalding had not yet arrived. As the trauma surgeon on call, it was his responsibility to be in attendance when surgery was performed by a resident. Jan tried calling him several times more but received no response. She considered calling the surgeon on second call, but was reluctant to cause any problems for Dr. Spalding. She checked to see how the surgery was going and waited. The patient had a ruptured spleen which had been removed and a lacerated liver that was being repaired. The patient was still losing blood and the residents were looking for additional sources of the bleeding. Almost three hours had elapsed when Dr. Spalding arrived. Jan began briefing him on the patient's status and noticed the unmistakable odor of alcohol. This was not the first time Dr. Spalding had arrived in the operating room smelling of alcohol when he was on call. He was known to have a drink or two but no one had ever questioned his operating skill. In fact, Jan had said "that if it were her or one of her family on that operating table there was no surgeon she'd rather have operating than Dr. Spalding." He was a superb teacher as well, and the residents consistently voted him "Faculty of the Year." In addition, he was well liked, confident, but never arrogant, and always considerate of the staff. The scrub nurses would volunteer to work overtime if it meant the opportunity to scrub for him.

But this Friday night was different. His speech was slurred and Jan knew he was drunk. She suggested they talk in the doctor's lounge, and once in there, she gave him coffee and told him she thought it best if he stayed in the lounge instead of scrubbing in. When she went back into the operating room, they were closing and the patient was stable. Jan breathed a sigh of relief and believed a crisis had been averted.

Saturday morning she received a call at home from the vice president for Nursing who had been contacted by a reporter from the local newspaper. He said he had information that emergency surgery had been performed last night on a critical patient by a physician in training because the surgeon showed up drunk. He was giving University Hospital an opportunity to comment before he contacted the patient's family. The story would appear in this afternoon's newspaper.

ETHICS ISSUES

Impaired Healthcare Professionals What is the responsibility of healthcare professionals related to impairment of themselves or others?

Adherence to Organization's Mission Statement, Ethical Standards and Values Statement Were the actions here consistent with the organization's mission statement, ethical standards and values statement? On the part of Jan Adams? On the part of Dr. Spalding?

Adherence to Professional Codes of Ethical Conduct Were the actions here consistent with the professional codes of conduct for physicians? For nurses? For resident physicians?

Legal Implications What is the hospital's liability for allowing a resident to perform surgery without the supervision of an attending physician? What is Jan's liability?

Management's Role and Responsibility As the operating room supervisor, what was Jan Adams' role and responsibility in this situation? What is senior management's responsibility following this incident?

Organizational Implications How will this incident be perceived by the public? What will be its impact on the organization?

Implications for Graduate Medical Education What are the implications of this incident on the surgical residency program? Should the program director for surgery education been notified?

DISCUSSION

Impaired Healthcare Professionals

Drug and alcohol abuse is a national reality with heavy social, financial, and ethical implications. The problem is much more serious in healthcare because of "the direct consequences of abuse by providers on the health and well-being of patients." As a result, the ethical obligations of colleagues, coworkers, and organizations related to substance abuse and those affected are considerable.[1] Substance abuse crosses all socioeconomic lines, but healthcare professionals have been found to be 30 to 100 times more likely to participate in substance abuse than the general population.[2]

Healthcare organizations, professional societies, and associations all have addressed the issue of drug and alcohol abuse and the impaired healthcare professional in ethical policy statements, codes of conduct, human resources policies, and the like. The American College of Healthcare Executives' Ethical Policy Statement on Impaired Healthcare Executives reminds us that impairment results in more than personal damage to the abuser and his/her family. It affects their organization, colleagues, patients, clients; their profession, their community, and society as a whole. Impairment typically leads to misconduct, incompetence, unsafe or unprofessional behavior, errors in judgment, and the like. The organization may suffer from a loss of public confidence and support. The College's policy statement defines ethical obligations of the healthcare executive including personal and professional behavior free of impairment, urging impaired colleagues to seek treatment, reporting them to the appropriate authorities if they do not, and recommending or providing resources for treatment within the organization and community.[3]

Adherence to Organization's Mission Statement, Ethical Standards, and Value Statements

The American Medical Association's Current Opinion of the Council on Ethical and Judicial Affairs focuses on the reporting of impaired colleagues. Noting that "physicians have an ethical obligation to report impaired . . . colleagues in accordance with the legal requirements in each state . . . to the hospital's in-house impairment program, if available . . . (or) the chief of an appropriate clinical service or the chief of the hospital staff . . . or directly to an external impaired physician program." It further notes that physicians who do not have hospital privileges should be reported to a physician impairment program such as those run by medical societies. If the physician does not enter an impairment program, then the physician should be reported directly to the state licensing board.[4]

The emphasis in both of these policies is treatment first, but each makes it clear that impaired professionals must be reported to the appropriate authorities if they do not enter treatment programs or continue to demonstrate impairment in professional activities. Given this direction, Jan should have reported Dr. Spalding to the chief of the department of surgery and Dr. Truman should have reported him to the program director for the surgery residency.

Progressive discipline for substance abuse is the norm in most healthcare organizations and many of today's healthcare organizations have Employee Assistance Programs (EAPs). The recovery rate for EAPs is 35 percent—60 percent of treated employees. The return is $4.23 for each dollar invested.[5] These are excellent statistics especially when you consider how much more costly it is to recruit, hire, and train a new employee. But EAPs are not always the answer. There is still some stigma attached to them, as well as the fear that entering such a program will damage one's career. Even though EAPs claim confidentiality, many avoid them for fear that their problem will become public. In addition, managed care insurance does not always cover the costs of an EAP program and employees may have to pay out-of-pocket.

Overwhelmingly, the most common workplace drug is alcohol and it is especially dangerous because supervisors and coworkers tend to overlook its abuse because it is not "illegal."[6] Coworkers may even rationalize misconduct on the part of a colleague by saying, "he was drunk at the time." Being drunk never justifies unethical, incompetent, or erratic behavior. Indeed, in a survey of Medical Group Human Resource Managers related to substance abuse in the workplace, 65.5 percent of those surveyed indicated that "people who hold the lives of others in their hands should be held to a stricter standard than others."[7]

Zetlin believes that an effective substance abuse program must have clear policies that have been developed through a collaborative process that determined why drug and alcohol use is unacceptable in the organization and what needs to be done about it. The collaboration should include representatives of human resources, legal counsel, safety departments, and the employees. If the organization is unionized, a representative of the union(s) should be included, as well. The program that is implemented must fit the organization, its culture and philosophy, and its business activity.[8]

It should include easy access to a reporting system that may function more effectively if it accepts anonymous information. As in the case at University Hospital, there may be great reluctance on the part of coworkers to report a colleague, especially if it is an individual they like and respect. They may not want to "get him/her in trouble" or hamper his/her career. They may be reluctant to report an impaired colleague for fear the persons may have privileges suspended, lose licensure, or be reported to the National Practitioner Data Bank. Concerned coworkers do not have many options when confronted with an impaired colleague. They may urge the individual to seek treatment or ask someone close to the individual to intervene. But if the impaired healthcare professional does not refrain from professional activity, the professional must be reported to protect the patients entrusted to the care of the organization.

Management's Role and Responsibility

In the case of nurses, J. K. Hall is clear on this point. "As professionals, nurses have a code which maintains that their *primary* ethical responsibility is to the patient."[9] In her book, *Nursing and Malpractice Risks: Understanding the Law*, Barbara Youngberg says that a nurse can be held personally liable if something goes wrong with a patient when a doctor does not respond to the nurse's call. If a doctor fails to respond to a nurse's call, the nurse should notify the nursing supervisor, the responsible hospital administrator, and the chair of the physician's department. The nurse's highest duty is to the welfare of the patient.[10]

Graduate Medical Education

The high quality of patient care for which teaching hospitals are known can be eroded if those hospitals do not conform to the highest ethical standards.[11] The public has been educated to believe that physicians in training are closely supervised by practicing physician specialists and subspecialists who are board certified in their field of specialty. Patient care thus takes place in an environment of intellectual inquiry which fosters the state-of-the-art practice of medicine.

When physicians in training perform unsupervised surgery, it invites mistrust of the institution and its healthcare professionals. When a faculty physician arrives in surgery intoxicated, it compounds this mistrust and further erodes the credibility of the institution that would allow such misconduct. Since teaching hospitals receive public benefits such as tax exemptions, training support, and research grants, they must do all they can to preserve the public's trust and confidence.

Organizational Implications

Stanley Reisor suggests that "institutions have ethical lives and characters just as their individual members do."[12] He cautions that the day-to-day interactions within a healthcare organization must reflect the values that it professes. To illustrate his point, he examines some of the contradictions that are often seen in academic health centers. Faculty may lecture medical students on the need to treat indigent patients the same as the insured and then turn the care of indigents over to residents; hospitals may build special facilities for the wealthy and ignore the poor in the neighborhood; faculty may instruct medical students to treat people with dignity while medical students are treated as nonpersons; administrators may call for cooperation while trying to undermine competitors. Reisor says that contradictions between what institutions say and what they do breeds cynicism among employees and staff and mistrust of the institution by society.[13]

In the case of University Hospital, the tolerance of Dr. Spalding's drinking alcohol while on call has not gone unnoticed by the operating room staff. Jan's failure to report him or to call the surgeon on second call has surely cost her the respect of her staff.

What about Dr. Truman and his responsibility as the resident in this case? Dr. Truman may be in a somewhat more precarious situation. Reisor reminds us that teachers and students are "bound together as family and subject to the ties that interdependence brings," and the regard for each other's needs should set the tone for them to follow ethical standards in their other healthcare relationships.[14] It would appear that this kind of teacher-student relationship would make Dr. Truman more vulnerable to compromising situations. That vulnerability is one of the reasons that there are policies in graduate medical education to help guide and protect physicians in training when confronted with situations such as these.[15] The accreditation bodies who review and accredit residency programs are interested in the policies and procedures that ensure sound educational practices and accreditation decisions impact the funding of residency programs. Dr. Spalding's behavior here is not just a personal matter, it is a program matter, as well. As a teacher, Dr. Spalding has a responsibility to serve as an ethical role model. In this case, he is teaching that "unsafe" patient care is acceptable.

Dr. Truman and Jan demonstrate misplaced loyalty in this case. As healthcare professionals, their primary loyalty should be with the patient. Codes of conduct for both the professions of medicine and nursing are clear on this. But both Jan and Dr. Truman like and respect Dr. Spalding's skill as a surgeon. This makes these kinds of decisions more difficult and also introduces the concept of fairness to the equation. Would Jan and Dr. Truman be as reluctant to report a surgeon that they did not like or respect? Probably not. Is this fair? Reisor tells us that fairness has a special significance in healthcare organizations for they cannot promote the equal valuing of all people and at the same time condone discriminatory practices.[16] When we like someone, we tend to show favoritism and sometimes overlook flaws that we would not overlook in others or we use their outstanding attributes to justify overlooking their flaws. Dr. Spalding may have a drinking problem but his contributions to the hospital and the teaching program are significant. This kind of rationalization can be dangerous as can the philosophy espoused by some that "all men are created equal; some are just more equal than others."

Notes

1. Worthley, J. A. 1999. *Organizational Ethics in the Compliance Context.* Chicago: Health Administration Press. 253.

2. Worthley, 261.

3. American College of Healthcare Executives' Ethical Policy Statement: Impaired Healthcare Executives, 1995.

4. American Medical Association, Current Opinion of the Council on Ethical and Judicial Affairs, 2000.

5. Worthley, 271.

6. Zetlin, M. 1991. "Combating Drugs in the Workplace." *Management Review* (Aug) 17–24.

7. Worthley, 273.

8. Zetlin, 17.

9. Hall, J. K. 1996. *Nursing Ethics and Law.* Philadelphia, PA: W. B. Saunders Co. 28.

10. Youngberg, B. 1996. *Nursing and Malpractice Risks: Understanding the Law.* Brockton, MA: Western Schools.

11. Conflicts in Academic Health Centers. 1990. Policy Paper: A Report by the AHC Task Force on Science Policy. Washington, DC: Association of Academic Health Centers. 25.

12. Reisor, S. J. 1994. "The Ethical Life of Healthcare Organizations." *Hastings Center Report* 24. No. 6. 28.

13. Reisor, 28–9

14. Reisor, 30.

15. Reisor, 32.

16. Ibid.

ETHICS ISSUES IN GRADUATE MEDICAL EDUCATION

Clinton H. Dowd, M.D.

INTRODUCTION

It is no surprise that there are ethical considerations in graduate medical education. The extent to which changes in the traditional paradigm for resident education have altered those considerations may be more revealing.

Classically, resident education has been carried out in university settings where a number of assumptions have been accepted:

1. Following the completion of their residency, candidates will leave to practice their craft elsewhere.
2. University-based teachers are rewarded on the basis of scholarly activity first and clinical practice second.
3. Post-residency fellows usually provide a significant amount of junior resident supervision as a "price" for the advanced education that they are receiving.
4. The departmental chairperson and the dean of the school control faculty monies, for the most part. The faculty thus works for a contracted amount plus incentives. This places tremendous control of faculty time in the hands of the leaders of the university.
5. Protected faculty time is used for the advancement of scholarly activity including the supervision of resident research. Research

faculty (nonclinical) enhances this environment and is supported by both private and governmental research grants.

6. Residency program directors are the departmental chairpersons although much of the daily supervision is delegated.

Over the last two decades a number of changes in this traditional paradigm have occurred. Historically, subspecialty care of major entities was rendered in the university setting with these cases being referred to the university medical centers from outlying regions. In an effort to provide this care, fellowships were granted to an ever-increasing number of residents finishing their training. This provided junior faculty support for the departmental clinical "grist mill" at minimal cost to the university and allowed the subspecialists to pursue their research and select clinical activity and academic careers in a relatively unfettered manner.

University Medical Centers, once a major source of pride and power for the medical schools, became a major financial drain as the federal government changed reimbursement from an "expense" formula to one based on "costs." The University Hospital faculty was forced out of their academic environment to compete for patient dollars from insurers. This competition was not limited to traditional university boundaries and soon the "battle was joined" between the university and the community medical centers.

Subspecialists were now much more readily available in the communities and community medical education moved away from the "poor step-child" where the residents were considered of insufficient caliber to be university residents and the faculty composed of only "generalists" who could not function without the assistance of the university specialty faculty.

For the subspecialty faculty who moved to the community setting, often with the threat of dire consequences such as not "passing" subspecialty boards, the clinical-oriented teaching environment was a marked financial bonus compared to the university stipends of their mentors. In many instances a reduction in research activity resulted due to the lack of formal fellowships, which were jealously guarded by the universities.

The university position was further eroded by the marked reduction in referrals from traditional nonuniversity medical centers. More and more the faculty was forced into direct competition for patient dollars with their referral sources. In the resultant university-community teaching system animosity could easily have been anticipated.

The ethical issues that will be dealt with in this essay are:

1. Resident recruitment
2. Resident evaluation

3. Resident retention and discipline
4. Faculty recruitment
5. Faculty discipline
6. Hospital administration and resident education
7. Research

RESIDENT RECRUITMENT

Residents for medical education programs are recruited from the allopathic and osteopathic schools across the country as well as from a large pool of international graduates, including those who are American citizens educated abroad as well as immigrants educated in other countries. The latter group often have gained access to the United States but may not have visas or work permits to allow them to easily enter the medical education stream.

Each education program serves a certain constituency of patients who ideally will have representation within the program. This may be difficult to achieve and if it is achieved, may have a long-term detrimental effect on the program.

For many years the residency review committee (RRC) collected statistics for each program as to the source of the residents. Programs that contained a surplus of candidates from sources that university programs did not traditionally employ were often viewed as "weak" and became subject to intense scrutiny from the RCC. The specialty boards routinely released information referring to "pass" rates by resident source (American Medical Graduate, Osteopathic Graduate, International Graduate, and U.S. International Graduate) which purported to indicate that one group performed at a higher level of function than another—regardless of the many considerations that played a part in that performance level.

The largest group of resident candidates come from the international pool. The response of individual programs to the almost overwhelming number of candidates has been quite consistent, particularly in programs that are viewed as being attractive to United States graduates. The applications are given at most a cursory evaluation because in-depth evaluation of the same level as U.S. graduates is impossible. Referees are unknown to the evaluators and thus the validity of the reference may be questioned. The examination system by which the candidate was evaluated is unknown or poorly understood. During the interview process, language skills may not be at the same level as that of American candidates. The result is that many popular programs do not evaluate all candidates on the basis of ability. The corollary is that less popular programs, either because of perceived undesirable locations (downtown, large, urban centers) or less popular specialties (e.g., psychiatry and anesthesia), have an overrepresentation of candidates perceived as being less desirable. The inference that the educational content of the program is not "up to standard" because of recruiting these residents, may place the program in jeopardy with the reviewing bodies.

Most residency programs will evaluate 10 to 15 candidates per position. A multitude of factors will be included in the consideration— past experience with candidates from the same educational institution, references (personal references are becoming a thing of the past with the RRC computerized application process), the program's experience with the individual (i.e., elective externships), the gender composition of the residency, the professional pressures that are brought to bear on the selection committee by administrators and colleagues seeking entrance to the program on behalf of friends, family, and acquaintances.

Few programs have a dedicated committee that will review all candidates, so final selections are usually made on a "point count" of various parameters as assessed by a nonuniform set of evaluators. Given the vagaries and uncertainties of the system, it is surprising that issues of beneficence and honesty can be satisfactorily addressed as often as they are.

Case 1:

A small program has the opportunity to recruit an international resident with impeccable credentials, but in doing so it will create a situation where the majority of residents are of international origin. Will this have a negative impact on subsequent recruitment of U.S. graduates? If a U.S. candidate is available, even if the credentials are not as good, should he/she be given preference? Their parents pay taxes which help to support the system, and their educational system which supports the residency programs needs to be able to "place" their candidates.

Case 2:

A group of international physicians lobby to have residents of their ethnic/religious origin given preferential treatment in the recruiting process so that their families will have specialists of similar backgrounds as treating physicians.

Case 3:

A resident candidate makes application to a program. The candidate has performed quite well on examination. This candidate falls under the guidelines of the Disabilities Act as a result of dyslexia and must be given extra time to accomplish assigned tasks. Should the candidate be granted equal consideration for a place in the residency program?

RESIDENT EVALUATION

Evaluation of the results of the education program need to be carried out on an ongoing basis so that candidates' progress up the learning curve can be plotted. This results in an evaluation of the candidate as well as an assessment of the quality of the teaching process. Some degree of standardization of the assessment is needed to create a "measure" by which all can be judged.

In-training examinations provide a standardized database assessment but are of little value in evaluating clinical judgment and competence. Written examinations created by the faculty have such a small denominator that they are of little statistical significance. The parameters of clinical judgment and competence must be assessed by the faculty. This, unfortunately, is extremely subjective and attempts to reduce these evaluations to a numerical constant have much less validity than many would like to believe. In general, these evaluations have the potential to degenerate into popularity contests involving both parties. Not many faculty are prepared to be the "bad guy" in the evaluation process.

As programs must now credential graduates, particularly in the technical areas so that they may receive hospital privileges, the validity of that process is of paramount importance. Failure of the process could potentially create significant medical-legal implications for the program and harm to patients.

Case 1:

A resident graduates from a program and in the course of a surgical procedure, causes irreparable harm to a patient. An ensuing legal action identifies that the residency program does not have documentation that the resident was capable of independently performing the procedure.

Case 2:

Upon the completion of the residency program, a candidate applies for specialty certification. Despite several attempts, the candidate fails to matriculate and as a consequence faces loss of hospital privileges and expulsion from HMO panels as a specialist. Suit is brought against the program for failure of its educational process to adequately prepare the candidate for the examination, and for the consequent ensuing financial loss to the graduate.

RESIDENT RETENTION AND DISCIPLINE

It would seem that all candidates, upon acceptance to the program, would identify successful completion of the residency as the highest priority. This is not the case. While most make the transition from medical student to resident physician with little difficulty, some struggle mightily with the change.

Although resident compensation is probably less than it should be, the increase in disposable income, compared to what the candidate was used to as a student, is significant. Quickly, life style changes occur: new cars, new spouses, new families, new social status, and some free time without the immediate pressure of impending examinations.

These factors conspire to distract the resident from what should be his/her primary goal—to get the most possible academic and technical information out of the program. In order to achieve this, the habits of reading and intellectual inquiry learned in medical school must be maintained and be honed. This has to occur in an environment where senior mentors often do not set a very good example—where the talk in the operating room is of last night's football score or the most recent fine wine that has been consumed. Harrison's *Textbook of Medicine* quickly seems to be pretty dull fare.

Not infrequently, new residents come from backgrounds where their families have not had the opportunities for education and success that the candidate is now experiencing. The resident has no background in how to function in the newly assumed role as a physician and cannot receive the degree of family support accorded many of their peers. This may create significant social pressure for the resident.

It is quite easy, despite an element of sleep deprivation, for the junior resident to perform his/her daily duties without much intellectual effort. Rounds are made with more senior residents and physicians who make most of the major decisions and plan subsequent evaluations and interventions. While some penetrating questions may be asked of the junior resident, more likely they will be directed to the medical student. By being cooperative in regard to the work output, (histories and physicals, order input) and being on time while looking neat and tidy for rounds, the junior resident can potentially "slide" for a period of time until a penetrating evaluation exposes the resident's lack of real progress as a physician. Like getting behind on taxes, this lost ground is very difficult to "make up," as new data acquisition rates must be maintained in the face of a deficit of information that has been allowed to occur.

While in many regards, this is the resident's problem, it is also the residency program's problem for several reasons:

1. A resident who cannot "carry his/her weight" places a greater burden on colleagues.

2. Greater effort must be spent by the faculty to remediate the resident, taking time away from other duties.

3. The resident suffers loss of status with his/her peers and faculty that may be difficult, if not impossible to recapture.

4. The resident suffers a major loss of confidence as a result of needing remediation.

5. The emotional impact of failure at this stage can be devastating for the resident. Severe depression and even suicide can result.

6. Resident recruitment suffers with resident failure and expulsion, as potential residents perceive that this might unjustly happen to them.

Once a resident has been identified as having significant deficiencies, these deficiencies must be corrected. Remediation must be accomplished within a reasonable time frame, but over enough time to allow adequate assimilation of the material in which the resident was deficient. Subsequent evaluation must confirm that the material has been mastered. If too long a time frame is allowed however, valuable time is lost in acquiring new material. If the remediation process is unsuccessful, the candidate has lost time in getting placed in an environment in which the resident can be successful.

If the remediation process is unsuccessful, major issues have to be dealt with. How much time should the resident be credited with within the program? Does the candidate have to be released from the program or can he/she be allowed to resign? What is the program's continuing responsibility to the resident and to any program that might subsequently hire the candidate?

These questions pose a serious concern to a program because, if the entire process is not clear cut and well documented, litigation will likely arise either on behalf of the former resident or on behalf of a patient alleging inappropriate treatment as a result of inadequate training.

Of at least equal concern is the consequence to the resident who has been dismissed—both personally as well as professionally. Will the resident be able to find a career in medicine that will be rewarding and allow the self-fulfillment that the resident sought on the first day of medical school?

In fairness to all, it must be realized that it is not just the deficient resident who is impacted in this process. Other resident colleagues have to pick up the slack. If dismissal results, can a replacement be identified who can fill the position so that call schedules, etc., are not permanently altered, perhaps putting the program out of compliance with the nationally mandated resident work hours.

If the resident does not receive credit for the time spent in a program, particularly a primary care program where the number of years of training is clearly laid out, Medicare funding to allow him to complete any program may be difficult to obtain. This raises the specter of either an uncompensated year or a year where a program would have to pay the resident stipend without remuneration from federal sources.

Case 1:

A resident in the second year of his program is confirmed as performing at an unacceptable level after taking the second year national training examination and achieving only the fifth percentile. The resident's performance earlier in the program had been marginal. The resident has received counseling in regard to the original performance. By the time that the results are available to the program, it is late March. Attempted remediation is completed three months later, but the subsequent examination results do not provide evidence of improvement. The ultimate decision to terminate the resident cannot be taken until September for a number of exceptional circumstances. Balance the action of dismissal between the impact on the resident and the impact on his fellow residents and the program.

Case 2:

Identify the duties that a residency program owes a candidate who is dismissed. Psychological counseling, job placement, another "chance," a favorable reference, or "no comment" to inquires from other programs?

FACULTY RECRUITMENT

Faculty recruitment has traditionally concerned, for the most part, subspecialists in a given field of endeavor. It has been anticipated that these individuals would perform research, provide their clinical expertise, and function as a traditional academic. Issues that were less germane included financial self-sufficiency, clinical supervision of non-specialty clinical care on a regular basis, and private practice.

The dramatic increase in the number of such specialists means that they now become a reality in the community medical centers, competing with their mentors at the universities for specialty cases and, because there may not be enough clinical demand for the subspecialty expertise in a small community, competing with the local generalists for private patient dollars while being subsidized by the local medical center.

While there has been a dramatic increase in the number of subspecialists, this increase pales in comparison to the amount of supervision of resident services that has been mandated by the federal government. Many of these subspecialty faculty, because of lack of current general experience, refuse to provide day-to-day clinical supervision beyond their "area of expertise." This refusal is partly fueled by the legal environment in which we live, partly because these individuals are "specialists," and partly because it interferes with the provision of private patient care for which they are very well remunerated.

In order to attract the subspecialists, faculty recruitment must involve generalists to provide supervision. The spiral of competition for private patient dollars thus continues at the less rarified atmosphere of the general patient. In order to successfully recruit young, enthusiastic generalists who are at the peak of their productivity, salary demands must be met and these are usually acceded to through supplementation of the salary with private practice dollars. The amount of federal contribution to faculty compensation is inadequate to support the amount of supervision that the federal government demands.

Attracting faculty to a residency program is even more demanding than recruiting residents, in regard to providing individuals who can be effective role models and teachers. These individuals will have a profound impact on recruiting, not only by their presence, but as well with their gender, ethnic, and racial backgrounds.

Just as ideally the resident group should, to some extent, reflect the patient populations that they serve, so should the faculty group. In this fashion, they role model appropriate patterns of behavior and demonstrate sensitivities that well may be lacking.

FACULTY RETENTION AND DISCIPLINE

Faculty employment opportunities at both university and community medical centers are extensive. In general, the community-based faculty have a greater interest in the provision of patient care. Opportunities for tenure tracks are infrequent in this setting and as a result the stimulus for research and academic writing is less rewarded than it is in the university setting.

The faculty in a nonuniversity setting, because salary from the institution represents a relatively small component of their stipend, tends to be harder to "control." There is no dean and the departmental chairman has relatively little authority except that to which the faculty voluntarily submit themselves. The financial control in this setting comes primarily from the hospital administration. These individuals may be poorly equipped to effectively referee this conundrum.

A reverse incentive exists for the faculty that possesses cutting edge technology to share this information with the residents in a community setting. Unlike the university setting, over 50 percent of residents trained in a community setting will remain in that setting to establish or join a practice. Trained in the advanced techniques, these new attending staff see little reason to refer their patients to the subspecialty staff who were their teachers for the specialized procedures. Consequently, the faculty are training their own competition. While teaching may be a stimulus for the faculty to maintain cutting edge technology, given the vagaries of funding these technologies, that stimulus may be more apparent than real.

A very real problem also exists with the retention and discipline of faculty in a community setting. The reasons that brought this valuable resource to the community are the very reasons that create the problem. While part of the motivation in coming to a community-based program was to teach and carry out research in a clinical setting, for most, an equally strong motivation was financial remuneration. This was balanced at the outset against the life style benefits and reduced clinical load at a university setting.

Creating a situation in the community setting that does not recognize the inherent differences in motivation for the community-based faculty will result in a system where faculty retention is impossible. Recruiting faculty and then losing them makes it virtually impossible to recruit replacements if the vacancy was created as a result of conflict.

Probably the most efficient way to solve the problem is for the medical center administration to delegate the control and negotiation of faculty contracts to the program director/departmental chairperson. Faculty physicians must ultimately be accountable to the medical center but otherwise the efficient management of this valuable resource is seldom achieved.

Case 1:

In the course of building a new subspecialty faculty division, a senior member of a university department is recruited as the divisional director. As the division grows, a junior is subsequently recruited. While both have excellent academic credentials, the junior physician strives to augment the divisional clinical activity without a complimentary increase in academic yield. Friction ensues and a split between the two physicians is inevitable. Hospital administration favors the junior physician due to the increase in clinical activity.

ADMINISTRATION AND MEDICAL EDUCATION

As hospitals have grown in size and complexity, there has been an increasing move to utilize professional managers who usually have little if any medical background. The professional managers, often endowed with credentials from prestigious business schools, bring to the educational setting a very different perspective than does the medical staff. The ultimate responsibility for the administrator may be fiscal viability and ensuring that the institution remains strong as compared to its competitors.

Traditionally, medical education was valued as a way to "give something back" to the training of medical staff, to enhance the prestige of the institution, and to serve as a catalyst for the medical staff to remain current. Currently, the nonteaching medical staff may play some mentoring role for residents and may provide some clinical supervision but these responsibilities are now all under the direction of the program director and staff.

As the residency program staff have taken over the supervision of the residency, the hospital administrative staff have accepted or taken over the responsibility for the fiscal viability of the programs. The faculty, needed for supervision and accreditation by the residency review committees, is often required to adhere to administration demands in order to generate their salary. In many cases, the salary contracts are created for faculty with little if any input from the program director. These contracts may well be contrary to the demands of quality resident education and frequently include time-consuming clinical duties, expanded programs outside the hospital, and nonteaching administrative responsibilities. Because the administration bears the ultimate financial responsibility for the institution, they tend to be loath to delegate contract responsibilities to the program directors whom they may view as fiscally less competent than they are. This administrative intrusion into the medical education program is understandable but it places the faculty in the position of working for two masters. It is a wise hospital administrator who can travel the rocky road of allowing the program director to manage his/her faculty in a fashion that fulfills the institution's needs and keeps the responsibility for residency education in the hands of physicians.

RESEARCH

No discussion of ethics issues related to graduate medical education would be complete without some mention of clinical research. Generally, there are three areas of concern where ethical dilemmas may present: 1) issues related to patient participants, 2) conflicts of interest, and 3) intellectual integrity. Issues related to patient participants surround informed consent, patient confidentiality, and most importantly, patient safety. Institutional review boards typically provide assurances that clinical trials and research studies are legitimate, appropriate and safe. Often less regulated are the areas of conflict of interest and intellectual integrity.

Much has been written about concerns related to the industrial funding of clinical research and how much influence this funding may have on the products of such research. Residency program directors and research staff must closely examine the methods that companies use to achieve their desired results. The study design, the study population, the comparable drugs and dosages used in the study, the time durations used to effectively demonstrate adverse effects, all impact the study results and must be appropriate. It has been implied that sometimes clinical investigators may be more interested in their personal financial gain than in the methods employed.[1] Conflicts of interest on the part of clinical investigators may be of special concern given the wide array of financial arrangements among hospitals, physicians, and suppliers to the healthcare field.

Equally as important are the issues of intellectual integrity. Who controls the data, who and where the results are published, and who authors the articles are all significant questions that left open may impinge on the integrity of the study results.

There are good reasons for teaching programs and the commercial sector to work together in research. Such collaboration provides enhanced income and resources for programs as well as opportunities for resident physicians. Program directors would be wise, however, to ensure that there are appropriate policies and guidelines in place to promote ethical standards of practice related to the conduct of all clinical research.[2]

Notes

1. Bodenheimer, T. 2000. "Uneasy Alliance: Clinical Investigators and the Pharmaceutical Industry." *New England Journal of Medicine* 342 (20): 1539–43.

2. Conflicts of Interest in Academic Health Centers, Policy Paper, A Report by the AHC Task Force on Science Policy. 1990. Washington, DC: Association of Academic Health Centers.

CHAPTER 5

WORKFORCE REDUCTION:
HILLSIDE COUNTY MEDICAL CENTER

Glenn A. Fosdick, FACHE

ILLSIDE COUNTY Medical Center is a 475-bed public teaching hospital located in an urban setting in the Midwest. It serves a city of approximately 250,000 people with a total county population of 500,000. Its primary local competition consists of two regional hospital systems, both not-for-profit. Due to its historical status as the county hospital and its urban location, it provides a significant portion (approximately 70 percent) of the uncompensated care for the community. Despite this, it receives no financial subsidies from the city or the county.

For many years, Hillside has been the primary tertiary center providing specialized care in high-risk obstetrics, a Level III neonatal intensive care program, and pediatric intensive and specialized care including pediatric oncology. In addition, Hillside is the regional provider for kidney transplants, burn services, and emergency medicine experiencing close to 80,000 visits per year to the ER. Hillside's services have been augmented over the last four years by the development of the region's first American College of Surgeons (ACS) verified trauma program. Hillside is affiliated with a major university medical school and has residencies in internal medicine, pediatrics, med/peds, and obstetrics and has a shared program with other hospitals in radiology and orthopedics. In addition, it has recently added an emergency medicine residency program.

Because it is a public hospital, Hillside has a board that is strongly committed to the community and to the medical center's mission. This has resulted in the development of a number of programs that have increased patient access and the capabilities of the hospital to meet its community health needs, including a large clinic providing primary and urgent care services in the most underserved area in the community. Unfortunately, due to the low reimbursement from outpatient Medicaid and the high percentage of uninsured that are served, the clinic experiences significant financial losses.

Like most hospitals, Hillside prospered until the mid-1980's when the changes in reimbursement and increasing competition began to impact it. In addition, Hillside is also heavily unionized with nine unions representing approximately 86 percent of its employees. This has resulted in higher than average benefit and pension costs. Because of multiple strikes and work actions during the 1980s, Hillside also found itself losing market share to its competitors. As its competitors grew stronger, Hillside started to face some significant financial challenges, which culminated in 1992 with a financial loss of close to $7 million. Through the recruitment of new leadership and enhanced strategic planning and marketing, the organization was able to correct itself and make significant progress. However, in the last several years, it has again faced increasing financial concerns. The dilemma it faces reflects the variety of problems that are common to most hospitals. These problems result from a number of specific issues, such as decreasing reimbursement, uncompensated care, increasing competition, volume, increasing costs, and personnel costs.

Clearly the most significant impact on national reimbursement resulted from the Balanced Budget Act of 1997 (BBA) or "BUBBA" as it is known in the healthcare field. Originally mandated to reduce Medicare expenditures by $116 billion over five years, "according to projections, the five-year impact of the BBA for hospitals and other Medicare providers is over $200 billion."[1] This alone has resulted in the loss to Hillside of approximately $13 million in revenue over the first three years of its implementation.

At the same time, the state in which Hillside is located has made a major revision in its Medicaid provision placing an increasingly high percentage of Medicaid care into a competitive Medicaid managed care environment. This has resulted in a reduction of cost to the state of approximately $300 million per year, which has been primarily felt by the

HMO's, hospitals, and physicians. Because Medicaid represents approximately 25 percent of Hillside's business, it has been adversely impacted by the reductions. Hillside serves a high percentage of uninsured and Medicaid patients and, thus, it is eligible for Disproportionate Share to Hospitals (DSH) payments. However, there have been increasing efforts to reduce these payments including the Balanced Budget Act of 1997.

Finally, Hillside is facing the difficulty common to all healthcare providers in actually receiving payment it is due for services that it provides. The financial pressures that insurers are facing appear to have encouraged them to find methodologies to make billing more difficult, to find justification for disqualification of bills, and in many circumstances to engineer significant delays in providing reimbursement for services that are properly billed. Although there have been some federal and state efforts to examine this issue, healthcare providers face unique challenges unknown in any other industry.

Paralleling national indicators, Hillside has seen an increase in the amount of uncompensated care it has provided over the last three years. Strategic analysis by the hospital suggests that locally this reflects to some degree the improving economy resulting in a population that disqualifies itself from Medicaid by taking entry-level jobs, which in many cases do not include health insurance. This is not a unique situation, for approximately 80 percent of the uninsured in the United States are employed. On a national basis, the uninsured population has grown since 1989 with 43.7 million Americans, 16 percent of the population, lacking insurance.[2]

In addition, Hillside is facing increasing challenges from nonhospital competitors in diagnostic and treatment areas that historically have been financially advantageous to the hospital such as, ambulatory, surgical, and diagnostic centers, including MRI facilities and dialysis centers owned and operated on a proprietary basis.

Like the majority of hospitals, Hillside faces the challenge of keeping its patient census as high as it has been in the past. Reductions in reimbursement for patients who stay longer than the appropriate time, increasing use of ambulatory services to treat patients in such areas as chemotherapy, surgery, and diagnostic scenarios, and increased competition from both regional and national sources have complicated Hillside's ability to maintain an average daily census.

At the same time, hospitals and other healthcare providers are experiencing dramatic increases in the costs associated with providing care. Drug expenditures have risen at a double-digit rate for the last four years. Medical/surgical and other supplies also continue to experience inflationary increases that exceed annual reimbursement adjustments.

Additional concerns are governmental mandates and accreditation standards, which require additional staff for nonpatient care requirements. For example, the recent implementation of the Federal APC outpatient billing system has necessitated additional coders to comply with increased mandates for medical record requirements.

Hospitals also face an intensely competitive environment for the recruitment and retention of healthcare personnel. Perhaps the most significant concern is the future availability of registered professional nurses. With a current average age of 44 years and a 20 percent reduction of new students entering nursing programs each year, there are valid concerns over the future availability of this critical portion of the healthcare system.[3]

This impending crisis also has specifically impacted the availability of nursing management staff. With increasing pressure for financial control and clinical improvement, there are a fewer number of qualified personnel interested in addressing these issues. Other shortages include, but are not limited to, ultrasound technicians, pharmacists, laboratory technologists, and radiation therapy personnel. All of this requires, on a very consistent basis, that Hillside reexamine its pay and benefit package to ensure that it is competitive and capable of attracting the right kind of personnel.

The increasing number of professional nursing staff that work for nurse staffing agencies is also a concern. These agencies allow the individual nurses to have increased control and independence over when and how many hours they work and to reduce vulnerability to required weekends and holiday coverage usually at the expense of benefits and pension plans. This contributes to a shortage of staff available to work these unattractive hours and the increased hourly rates result in additional costs to hospitals such as Hillside.

Difficulties in recruiting nurses and the financial requirements of tight staffing have also increased the need for overtime and mandatory overtime. In addition to higher costs, concerns over the strain on staff and the impact excessive overtime has on the quality of clinical care has attracted interest from state legislatures to develop controls regarding the use of overtime. Increased overtime also stimulates reaction from unions which can result in strikes and other work actions.

These combined pressures have resulted in the difficulties that are presently being faced at Hillside. As the CEO and the management staff sit down to examine their situation, it becomes very clear that unless significant changes are made quickly, Hillside's financial viability will be compromised. The CEO also recognizes that these issues are more important today than before. His board, like many, has increasingly identified the operating margin and profitability and financial perfor-mance as the primary indicator of the contribution of the management team.

In addition, due to the size and complexity of healthcare capital expenses today, there is an increasing dependence on the bond market, which puts great significance on bond ratings from recognized financial assessment organizations. A change in an organization's bond rating will have a significant effect on its ability to borrow long-term capital and on the cost of that capital.[4] The CFO has made it very clear that a reduction of the hospital's bond rating is possible and could significantly increase costs in the area of capital finance. He has pointed out that in the past year the number of hospitals that have received lower bond ratings has increased at approximately five times those that have been upgraded.

The CFO also notes that in previous discussions with rating agencies, the agencies have now implemented a new definition for hospitals called the "Century Club." This dubious distinction pertains to those health-care organizations that have lost at least $100 million in the previous year. In the past several years, there have been at least a dozen institutions that have met this qualification.

Accordingly, the CEO, recognizing the critical importance of swiftly and properly addressing these financial concerns, called his senior man-agement staff together. He has decided that because of the need to address this issue from a corporatewide viewpoint, it is essential that all senior management personnel be involved to ensure the best results.

Because of the financial significance, the CFO takes the initiative. He notes that, as in most healthcare organizations, the highest portion of expense is associated with staff. Under the present salary and benefit package, for example, the average employee costs Hillside approximately $45,000 per year. He indicates that even with the cost of unemployment liabilities and potential severance programs, reductions in the workforce are the safest and best known method of reducing financial deficiencies.

The vice president for Human Resources reminds the group that in most union contracts and many state labor codes, seniority is a key determinant in the reduction of staff. At Hillside for example, the present contracts in key unions such as nursing stipulate that seniority is determined on a hospitalwide basis. He notes that the least senior nursing staff may be located in critical areas such as the emergency de-partment and operating rooms where their services are essential for con-tinuing financial productivity. He also states that with multiple unions, comparative numbers affected from each union as well as the ratios of reduction to management personnel are monitored very closely and could have implications on labor stability.

The vice president for Nursing and the vice president for Medical Affairs collectively announce that patient care cannot be compromised and that inappropriate reductions in these areas could have a critical impact on the clinical capability and reputation of the organization. Finally, the vice president for Operations questions the impact on community projects such as the clinic and whether there are other approaches that might be taken. It is these questions that the CEO ponders as he contemplates the right approach to successfully address these issues.

As the CEO examines these financial challenges, he tries to identify the dynamics of the healthcare industry that separate it and make it distinct from other industries. While it is true that other industries have faced the need for reductions in the number of employees, there may be no other environment that incorporates the multifaceted responsibilities of the healthcare institution. Certainly financial performance, while important, is not the only criteria that must be measured. The CEO knows that Hillside must ensure that adequate and proper care is provided and available to those who seek it. There is no other business he can think of where a person receives the service, in many cases, prior to identifying how payment will be provided for that service. Recent mandates from the federal government, in fact, prohibit assessment of financial status prior to providing emergency medical care.

In addition, Hillside's mission clearly defines its responsibilities to improve the health of the community. Because the vast majority of hospitals in the United States like Hillside have either not-for-profit or public tax status, they are required to provide services in some cases that are contrary to normal business standards. Unfortunately, the public perception too often is that this requirement is not being met.

The CEO reminds himself that a recent survey performed in 1998 by the American Hospital Association indicated that the general public was losing confidence that hospitals were fulfilling this requirement and has begun to equate them with drug companies and defense attorneys. The CEO felt strongly that Hillside must live up to its mission and he knew that as a public hospital there would be close scrutiny to see that it did.

ETHICS ISSUES

Organizational Implications What is the appropriate and most ethical method of addressing the potential financial shortcomings of the organization? Who should the CEO listen to as he determines the appropriate course of action? Should he include others beyond senior management? If so, who?

Adherence to Hospital's Ethical Standards and Values In identifying the best approach, does it reflect and adhere to the responsibilities of the mission of the organization? How does the CEO prioritize financial viability with clinical quality, organizational mission and community responsibilities?

Management's Role and Responsibility Is rightsizing the only answer or even the best answer to addressing financial difficulties? Does it ensure that the impact and exposure to these difficulties are shared across all levels and groups within the organization? Is this possible while accomplishing the financial and clinical needs? Should the CEO be examining other options that may also address the organizations financial concerns? Does the approach ensure that the effect of the decision does not create more difficulties in the long run than the decision itself?

Clinical Quality Should the decisions on cutbacks be determined from a clinical viewpoint or a business viewpoint?

DISCUSSION

Participation in Problem Resolution

A fundamental question is who should be participating in the resolution of this problem? While it is true that the CEO has sought input from the key members of his senior management staff, is that adequate?

A unique characteristic of a hospital is the significance of the stakeholders involved with and influenced by its actions. With a problem of this magnitude, should they be involved and as importantly, can they help? To decide this, it is first necessary to identify who they are, how they may be affected, and what may be the potential positive and negative ramifications of their involvement.

Medical staff. Because of their dominant role in the hospital as a customer, provider of care, leader, and political force, it is most appropriate to start with the medical staff. Because any changes in staffing or services will directly influence the care provided to *their* patients, concerns regarding these issues are to be expected and understood. In addition, because they have evolved as an informal (and sometimes formal) representative for hospital staff, it is to be expected and assumed that they will hear all the rumors (often inaccurate) and fears of the staff and in many cases, will attempt to defend and protect them. Such efforts may include discussion with board members or utilization of the formal medical staff structure to react to any considered changes or reductions. Because it is difficult to do rightsizing without impact on services, medical staff concerns in some circumstances may be quite legitimate. More importantly, the medical staff can be of value in determining how and what to do in addressing this problem.

The CEO must understand that the medical staff will be affected and will be a part of this process in some way. It can be defensive and disruptive or it can be collaborative. Due to the unfortunate common-ality of financial problems in healthcare, staff reductions are no longer unthinkable to members of the medical staff. Accordingly, the CEO has the opportunity to identify this challenge as one that requires the combined efforts of the medical staff and management. To accomplish this, the CEO must attempt to educate and share his concerns with the medical staff in a variety of settings. The use of the formal structure beginning with the medical executive committee is beneficial. However, informal discussions at departmental meetings or with key individual physicians is essential.

It is important to remember that the medical staff has the capacity to contribute greatly towards the resolution of this problem. Reductions in length of stay, usage and selection of medical/surgical supplies, and increases in admissions are possible and may be prioritized as an alterna-tive to losing popular staff or important services. Finally, involvement in these tough decisions may enhance the medical staff's appreciation that after thorough analysis, what is done is unfortunately the most feasible approach available.

Governing board members. Although it is obvious that the board will be involved in the formal approval stages of this process, it is also important to consider the value they may provide in the decision phase as well. Recognizing the diverse backgrounds that a board may represent and the increasingly common experience that other industries have in rightsizing, it is very possible, if not probable, that this may be an area where they are experienced. The CEO must be willing to utilize all available expertise in his attempt to accomplish any staff reductions with the least negative impact. It is also important to note that the more involved the board is, the greater support that will be received on this matter and the better prepared board members will be to respond to any personal inquires they may receive regarding actions.

Unions. Although historically unions were more common in public hospitals, the representation by unions nationally is increasing dramatically. For example in 1997, an all time high of 197 union petitions were filed with the National Labor Relations Board (NLRB) and this trend continued to rise even higher with 203 petitions filed in 1998. As significantly, the win rate (61.7 percent in 1998) was significantly higher then in general industry.[5] The increasing involvement of unions has also required the development of new skills for senior managers to successfully work in a union environment.

Although the most common approach utilized by American management in planning rightsizing is to notify unions of the plan for reductions, the CEO should strongly consider the involvement of union leadership in the process at an earlier time. The ability to "share" this problem and identify it as an issue common to all parties may focus the negative feelings away from the hospital and management and concentrate them on the external forces that are causing the financial problems. In addition, it is important to recognize the value of input that may be gained from union leadership.

The CEO recalls hearing of one organization in similar circumstances that spent over 30 hours in one week with key union leaders examining the entire operating budget and seeking feedback on each line item. From this, management was able to implement a number of sound ideas for reducing costs that they may not have perceived on their own. As importantly, the experience demonstrated to union leadership the difficulty that management was facing and their efforts to reduce costs in the best and fairest manner possible.

Essential to the success of this approach with union leadership and employees is the following:

- Initial cuts must first be made at the level of vice president, associate administrator, or senior departmental director.
- No particular department or segment of the organization should be exempt from rightsizing, unless completely justifiable.
- If at all possible, an equal percentage of managers should be dismissed in proportion to an equal amount of employees.
- Managers should exhibit and communicate to their employees the sacrifices they are making as a result of the rightsizing. For example, managers should indicate the lack of available resources in the financial budget, a lack of personnel, or other detrimental conditions caused by the rightsizing, so employees understand that there is no difference between the effect of rightsizing on managers and employees.[6]

These actions will allow union leadership to return to their respective constituents with a strong appreciation of the challenge involved and the intent of management to address it fairly. This appreciation could also be important when considering how union leadership may respond to the media. In many cases, hospitals can experience criticism of their ability to provide adequate and safe care after a reduction in workforce. This may result in a further reduction in volume and the need for additional cost and staff reductions. However, if union leadership has participated in the process and is comfortable that the actions were truly required, were fairly and consistently executed, and the commitment of the institution remains on patient focus, it is possible to have an appropriate and supportive response from union leadership.

Employees. Progressive and beneficial feedback from employees in this area is also possible. Providing employees with the opportunity to identify cost-saving options, educating them on what will happen if costs cannot be reduced, and incorporating them into the process where possible has the potential to identify new approaches and to avoid mistrust of management. Communication with employees is critical as the issue develops. Rumors, misinformation, and anger toward management are not beneficial and are traditionally disruptive and counterproductive.

It is the responsibility of the CEO to define guidelines that ensure that all staff resources are incorporated into the process even over the recommendations of members of management who prefer to make these decisions the "easy way." Fear of politically impacting the process and delaying needed reductions is common and while having merit, this is not the time for management to be autocratic.

If properly managed, rightsizing can lay the foundation for a new, vibrant organization. If poorly managed, it can become perhaps the singularly most dangerous threat to organizational survival and a major cause for employee turnover and destruction of organizational morale; at its worst, rightsizing can cause the demise of the heretofore successful healthcare organization.[7]

Exploring Other Options

A critical issue of rightsizing is the determination that it is the right and/or the only approach to address the organization's financial difficulties. A common phenomenon experienced is the premise that the desired goal is reducing costs. That is not accurate. The primary goal is to improve overall financial viability. The organization will be measured on its financial viability and it is important to its long-term success.

The CEO should remember that if cutting costs were the only goal, then closing all the nursing units would be extremely effective. A huge percentage of costs will be reduced. However, the loss of revenue will obviously override that approach. Improvements in financial viability can be accomplished via two avenues: reducing costs and increasing revenues. All too frequently the focus in healthcare has been directed toward cost reduction.

Although the overall high costs of the healthcare industry certainly support this interest, it is not always the most beneficial direction for the organization and the community it serves. The CFO often prioritizes a cost reduction strategy for several good reasons:

1. It is clearly the fastest method of addressing financial concerns.
2. It is, in the short run, the most reliable and measurable. As previously stated by the CFO, even when incorporating the unemployment and severance separation costs, the savings are well defined and expedient.
3. It certainly may have some justification. It is commonly difficult not to have the costs of care increase and exceed reimbursement in healthcare today.

However, it is the role of the CEO to recognize cost reduction as only one option and ensure that all possibilities are explored for the long-term success of the organization.

For example, in the case of Hillside Hospital, one possible opportunity may be review of its public status. Although the transformation of a public hospital to a not-for-profit may be publicly difficult and expensive, it is an option that has frequently been utilized in the last decade. There are some distinct financial advantages and some potential disadvantages associated with a move of this type. Public hospitals in many states are constrained on their ability to invest cash reserves, which over the last several years in the highly productive financial market resulted in significant limitations on potential returns from these investments. In addition, elimination of the public hospital status may enhance the ability of the hospital to refine its benefit or pension status to a more competitive one that is parallel to those of not-for-profit hospitals. On the negative side, losing public status could reduce Hillside's access to certain Disproportionate Share Payments and other potential benefits that have been identified for public hospitals. In this example, all aspects should be reviewed and examined to determine the value and potential impact of this transformation.

The organization should also examine the potential for reducing or eliminating clinical programs within the hospital itself. Although historically the strategic approach has been to provide as many different services as possible, it has become obvious in the recent past that maintaining programs with decreasing volume and expensive qualifications and support needs may not be beneficial. Collaboration with other providers does not require the closing of services or clinical loss to the community.

Collaborative efforts between organizations may allow agreements that result in services being reduced in one facility in return for a service being dropped at another. Both facilities may expand their volume and potentially increase their profit margin. It is imperative in this case that the CEO and senior management not be limited by historical protocol. A fact that other hospitals have "always provided" certain services does not preclude them from change. A progressive and well-planned effort to reduce duplication of services and commit to their provision by one provider may be well received by insurers, local industry leaders, and the community as well. While it is naive not to assume that there may be some concerns voiced by physicians and staff presently providing these services, this may be minimal compared to the continued reduction of overall capability within your institution.

Revenue Enhancement

The competitive environment of healthcare today has made identifying additional opportunities to expand revenue increasingly challenging. Efforts should revolve around several key areas:

A. Ensuring that payment is received on a timely basis and at the highest amount for services rendered. Opportunities in this area include reviewing the present billing system to identify departmental performance. This assessment includes at minimum:

1) *Days in receivables (compared to state and national averages)*: Changes in performance over the last 24 months may also identify problems that are increasing or have evolved in the recent past.

2) *Charge rates*: An external review of charge rates may identify possible areas of improvement particularly in areas such as operating rooms and ambulatory facilities.

3) *Analysis of individual insurance agreements*: This may allow consideration of renegotiation of contracts or consideration of separation from certain contracts.

4) *Internal analysis of charging programs*: This will ensure that charges are developed on a timely basis for all services rendered.

B. Review of patient volume to ensure that the highest volume of patients is obtained for each service rendered:

1) An in-depth inspection of admission rates by physician and service, combined with a yearly analysis of market share data will help identify changes or opportunities in volume and provide information for the CEO to discuss with the medical staff and help identify strategic priorities for the recruitment or placement of new physicians. The CEO should also examine the ages of the medical staff to identify needs for future recruitment.

2) An analysis of patient satisfaction scores is important as it may clarify additional reasons why patient volume is being affected. Recognizing the competitive environment may require a clear assessment of the present facilities and a commitment by staff to enhance customer service.

3) New and additional service opportunities are explored in depth to identify all available revenue sources. The CEO should examine each of these areas in great detail with the appropriate staff. It should be noted that due to the competitive nature of healthcare today, finding options for new revenue-producing programs is not easy. The proverbial low-lying fruit have probably been picked and new programs may require significant investment and/or a time delay before profits are accomplished. However, it is essential to recognize that this is a key responsibility of the CEO in order to move the organization forward.

It should also be noted that to make investments of this type at this time will require the confidence of the board and the medical staff and may be criticized by union leaders or other employees. It is the responsibility of the CEO to keep these important stakeholders focused on the vision for the long-term success of the organization and to assist other stakeholders to appreciate that this is not a short-range crisis but rather an industry direction.

Clinical Quality

A major issue facing the CEO is determining if any contemplated rightsizings will impact on the quality of the organization's clinical care. The nature of the industry requires decision makers including the board, CEO, and senior management to appreciate the necessity and lack of flexibility available when it comes to quality issues.

At no recent time has this been under more scrutiny then today. The Institute of Medicine report, *To Err is Human*, indicated in 1999 that the results of two significant studies "imply that at least 44,000 and perhaps as many as 98,000 Americans die each year as a result of medical errors." The report also noted that medication errors are costly to the institution citing a recent study that found "about 2 percent of admissions experienced a preventable, adverse drug event resulting in increased hospital costs of $4,700 per admission."[8] As a result of this report, significant efforts are underway on the part of the federal government to monitor quality concerns through the Health Care Financing Agency (HCFA). In addition, accrediting agencies including the Joint Commission on Accreditation of Healthcare Organizations (JCAHO) have also identified specific, new, and expanded requirements that pertain to clinical quality issues.

At the same time, private industry is banding together in a manner and at a level never seen before to establish new guidelines and mandates for healthcare providers. The Leapfrog Group represents over 60 national corporations with 20 million employees who represent an annualized health insurance cost of over $60 billion. In November of 1999, it released its plan "to have employers agree to base the purchase of healthcare on principles encouraging more stringent patient safety measures. These measures include: 1) computerized physician order entry, 2) evidence-based hospital referral, and 3) intensive care unit (ICU) staffing by physicians trained in critical care medicine."[9]

These efforts require the CEO to analyze each move in a rightsizing effort to make certain that the organizational clinical quality is not compromised. The challenges associated with the expanding demands of clinical capability and reducing reimbursement do not excuse the organization from performance at an acceptable level of quality. To do so requires a new level of understanding and utilization of information and a collaborative working relationship with the medical staff, nursing leadership, and senior management. It may result in a series of short-term decisions that define the ability of the organization to provide an acceptable level of care one day at a time.

Community Health

At the same time, the organization's capabilities to maintain their commitment to community health programs must be given priority. These assessments should take into account potential for improved health and efficiencies as well as the contemplation of reduction in programs. The CEO at Hillside must, for example, carefully examine the clinic providing care to the underserved population. At a time when the organization's overall future viability is at stake, it is possible that it may be determined that programs of this type are unaffordable. In many cases, programs of this nature may incur front-end financial losses but may also reflect significant admissions and laboratory and diagnostic tests that add financial value to the organization. It is imperative that the entire financial contribution of a program of this type be examined to determine its true bottom-line impact on the organization. Identifying what will happen if this program is not in operation is also valuable. If its patients, for example, are required to then utilize the emergency room resulting in increased overcrowding and delays in getting admissions and care provided to the more emergent patient; this has a very real potential cost.

Finally, it is imperative to examine what other options might be available to retain a valuable program of this type. Is it possible, for example, to share the costs of this program with other healthcare providers? Are there grants or governmental funds that may provide support for a program of this type that contributes to the overall health of the community? Is there a federally funded health clinic in the community that could take over the operation of the Hillside clinic and make it eligible for financial support?

It is important to understand that there are also the political costs associated with closure of a program of this type. Underserved communities have become extremely sensitized through their experience of having services reduced or eliminated and it is not uncommon for them to react with criticism through the media, to community leaders, or in other ways such as picketing. These concerns must be addressed when contemplating the true cost of reduction of these services.

Collaboration

Financial challenges provide an opportunity for organizations like Hillside to examine the possibility of increased collaboration with competitors. Because of the universal nature of the financial difficulties being experienced by healthcare organizations, it is quite probable that competitive hospitals are experiencing these challenges as well. In these circumstances, there may be opportunities to work collectively and merge certain services to avoid duplication, reduce costs, and enhance the overall quality of programs provided. Opportunities may include programs such as jointly run MRI or other radiological test centers, centralized laboratory systems, and support services such as laundry, freestanding security services, and ambulance services. In addition, this opens up the opportunity for strategic assessment of programs that are consistent between hospitals and possible collaboration.

This may be accomplished through a joint operating agreement, which allows both institutions to collectively work together and share the benefits saved by avoiding duplication. An agreement reached by Hillside with Behavioral Medicine Services that resulted in the closure of a freestanding outpatient behavioral center of one facility and the closure of the inpatient pediatric adolescent unit of the other is an example. The end result was significant savings and improved utilization by both parties.

Leadership

The financial problems experienced by Hillside Hospital have become common in the health industry over the last decade. Decreases in revenue, increases in cost, and reductions in inpatient volume have required institutions like Hillside Hospital to deal with significant threats to their financial viability, in many cases requiring immediate action and tough decisions. To some degree, this has moved the healthcare industry closer in parallel to other industries in the United States. No longer is the healthcare system a stable industry that does not experience layoffs and reduction in force as it was in the past.

These new challenges require healthcare administrators to become better leaders and more sophisticated managers capable of making tough decisions. These financial challenges combined with the expansion of healthcare unions, managed care, and increasing pressure on physicians have made it imperative that healthcare administrators develop the skills necessary to work collaboratively with medical staff, union leaders, and employees. They must enhance their ability to lead the institution in the strategic planning process, take the strategic vision that evolves, sell it to the primary stakeholders, and make it work. Once key services are defined, they must have the ability to monitor and measure these programs to determine if and when they need enhancements or reductions. Recognizing their obligation to community service, they must find a way to ensure that successful programs can pay for those that are less financially attractive.

As changes take place and outside influences impact the industry, health services administrators must lead their institutions in the correct direction to cope with them. In the last five years there have been multiple examples where actions of external decision makers have had unforeseen impact on organizations. For example, as government has encouraged the closure of hospital beds, they have ignored what takes place in the hospital's emergency services. Through the reduction of reimbursement for home and long-term healthcare, over 25 percent of the home health agencies in the United States have closed over the last several years and many long-term care providers are having significant financial problems. Little consideration was given to the negative impact of the inability of the hospital to discharge patients and to control length of stay. Little consideration was given to unexpected and nonproductive increases in costs associated with the Y2K adjustments, HIPPA, and the APC Medicare Outpatient Reimbursement System. It is the responsibility of the CEO to successfully and ethically address these challenges without compromising the clinical care provided by his institution.

Although there are many parallels to other industries, there are significant differences placed upon the expectations for providers of healthcare. It is difficult to move a hospital to another community because of the possibility of reduced costs and still have the hospital fulfill its mission. It is unethical, ill advised, and illegal to turn away patients requiring emergency care due to their financial status. As healthcare executives deal with these challenges, it is hoped that they do so in a more compassionate way than some other industry leaders. The willingness of large corporations to cut tens of thousands of jobs to enhance the profit margins to their stockholders is well known. It is hoped that as healthcare executives deal with their financial concerns that they start by looking in the mirror and asking themselves whether they have done everything possible to effectively reduce costs, improve financial performance, and enhance the product to make it more attractive to consumers. If they cannot convince themselves of this, it is imperative that they do not take the easy way out and comfortably cut staff. The ability to deal with these issues will separate the successful and ethical administrator from the pack.

Notes

1. American Hospital Association, Impact of the Balanced Budget Act of 1997 on Providers and Patients, Report before the Commerce Subcommittee on Health and Environment of the United States House of Representatives (July 19, 2000).
2. Lascinski, R. 2001. "2nd Analysis, The Alarming Growth in the Number of Uninsured." [Online information retrieved 2/15/2001]. www.drkeop.com
3. Carpenter, D. 2000. *Going, Going, Gone, Hospital and Health Network*. Chicago: American Hospital Association. 33.
4. Gapenski, L. C. 1996. *Understanding Healthcare Financial Management*. Chicago: AUPHA Press. 215.
5. Adams, W. 2000. "Why the Healthcare Industry Should Fight Union Organization and the High Cost the Industry Will Pay if Its Fight Is Unsuccessful." *Healthcare Manager* 18(4): 8–9.
6. Lombardi, D. N. 1997. *Reorganization and Renewal: Strategies for Healthcare Leaders*. Chicago: Health Administration Press. 42.

7. Lombardi, 53.

8. Committee on Quality of Healthcare in America, Institute of Medicine. 1999. *To Err Is Human, Building a Safer Health System.* Washington, DC: Nation Academy Press.

9. The LeapFrog Group for Patient Safety. 2000. "The Business Roundtable Launches Effort to Help Reduce Medical Errors Through Purchasing Power Clout." [Online information retrieved on 11/15/2000].
http://www.leapfroggroup.org/PressEvent/PressRelease.pdf

LEGAL PERSPECTIVES

Walter P. Griffin

"Illegal actions may be unethical. Unethical actions may be legal."

Anonymous

LTHOUGH THE general public may view military intelligence and ethical lawyers as oxymorons, in the field of healthcare the lawyer must be aware of not only the legal implications, but the ethical implications, in representing healthcare professionals. Although unethical behavior may not be illegal per se, a fine line exists between the two disciplines which can be easily crossed. It is the responsibility of a lawyer to guide his client along the line of demarcation by differentiating among illegal actions, unethical actions, and appropriate actions.

As debated throughout this book, these definitions and the lines separating the clients' behavior are not always obvious. Lawyers are continually taught by their experiences in courtrooms that debate and court rulings establish the separation between illegal actions, unethical actions, and appropriate actions and reinforce that the areas of separation are fluid and subject to continual change. A legal opinion elicited from any attorney on a Tuesday could be altered, voided, or confirmed by a court of competent jurisdiction when the same issue is raised in another case later that same week. The ebb and flow realized from multi-jurisdictional decisions continually modifies and alters opinions given by lawyers. The timing of lawyers' opinions is crucial. An opinion promulgated in one year may not have any force or effect in the next year. Although it seems improbable that legalities and ethical behaviors can continually be modified and varied, this occurs historically.

UNIVERSITY HOSPITAL

In the University Hospital case scenario, the basic principles are definable but the actions required by the participants, stemming from those principles, are less definable. A second-shift supervisor for the OR, who has great respect for the attending trauma surgeon, was placed in a position between well-founded underlying legal principles and a variety of actions which could be taken based upon those principles. The underlying legal principles are: the second-shift supervisor for the OR has an independent legal duty to stop the intoxicated trauma surgeon from performing surgery; and a legal duty to contact the second-call trauma surgeon when the original trauma surgeon did not arrive in a timely manner to assist the resident in lifesaving surgery. Besides these legal duties, a strong argument can be made that the second-shift supervisor, in her managerial capacity, has an ethical duty to report the intoxication of the trauma surgeon to her superior. The ethical responsibility is to the community at large.

It can also be argued the nurse supervisor had a legal obligation to report the incident since the hospital is responsible, on the theory of respondent superior, for the action of a trauma surgeon supplied by the hospital in an emergency situation. It does not make a difference whether the surgeon was an employee of the hospital or was acting as an independent agent.

Another issue is whether the nurse supervisor had a responsibility to stop the resident from performing surgery. Assuming the resident had a license to practice medicine within the state where the University Hospital is located, the nurse supervisor did not have the legal responsibility to stop the resident from performing surgery. However, the nurse supervisor may have had a legal responsibility to notify the patient's relatives that life-threatening surgery was being performed by a resident, to obtain permission to proceed since the patient was unconscious, and then to contact the second-call trauma surgeon because of the delay or the inebriation of the original trauma surgeon when he arrived. By obtaining consent from the patient's relatives and by notifying the second-call trauma surgeon, both the ethical and legal obligations have been discharged. For the nurse supervisor to take any other action from these underlying principles exposes the hospital to liability for allowing a resident to perform surgery, even though it may be justified under the emergency situation, and certainly exposes the hospital to liability for the failure of the nurse supervisor to notify the second-call trauma surgeon when no supervising trauma surgeon was present. The hospital, in all likelihood, would not be responsible for the intoxicated trauma surgeon since he did not perform the surgery and if the hospital was unaware of any previous episodes of intoxication.

With respect to the actions of the resident, it is assumed the resident was licensed to practice medicine within the state where the University Hospital is located and, therefore, the resident has not violated licensing laws. Concerning the legality of performing surgery, it is presumed that a licensed resident can practice medicine and surgery under the statutes of the state. However, whether or not the resident is competent to perform the surgery in question creates legal exposure for the University Hospital. The question would be whether the resident, under the procedures and regulations of the hospital, has privileges to perform surgery, and from an ethical standpoint, whether the life-threatening condition of the patient demands action whether or not the required privileges had been extended to the resident. Clearly, the resident relied upon the fact that an attending physician would be present to legitimize the resident performing the surgery. The attending physician's presence would have been mandatory if the necessary privileges had not been extended to the resident. But the ethical considerations in this case remain the same. Ethically, the resident must intervene. The resident's personal liability may be abrogated by the defense that a life-threatening emergency demanded intervention with or without the extension of privileges or the annointment of competency. However, the resident should have instructed the nurse in charge to call the second-call trauma surgeon. The resident should also have notified the residency program director of the intoxication of the trauma surgeon in the interests of safe patient care in the future.

PARADISE HILLS MEDICAL CENTER

A basic legal principle is established in the Paradise Hills Medical Center oncology program "misadventure." Clearly, the hospital is responsible for the actions of its employee, that is, the medical physicist whose calculations allowed excessive levels of radiation to be administered to 22 oncology patients.

The legal and ethical questions here are whether the institution has an obligation to notify the patients of the mistake, even though the results of the mistake may not adversely affect the patients; whether the ordering physician should be informed of the mistake and that physician allowed to decide whether the patient should be notified; or for the hospital management to simply do nothing. From a legal point of view, the doctrine of fraudulent concealment is important. An institution or physician who withholds medical information from a patient, which may be detrimental to that patient, may have established the basis for a claim of fraudulent concealment. An easier example is, a surgeon who knows a sponge has been retained in a patient after surgery and does not tell the patient of the retention of the sponge, has fraudulently concealed a fact upon which a lawsuit could be formulated.

In the Paradise Hills Medical Center instance, each patient who received an excessive dose of radiation has a cause of action. The cause of action would be based upon medical negligence. To fraudulently conceal this information would not only establish a separate cause of action, but would indefinitely extend the statute of limitations which might otherwise bar such action. Therefore, to legally conform, the patients should be notified. This notification also satisfies the ethical implications.

There is, however, one more decision. Is it the responsibility of the institution or the ordering physician to notify the patients? The institution may discharge its legal obligations by notifying the ordering physician of the error on the theory that the physician is acting as the outer ego of the patient, but the ethical responsibility of the hospital may indeed have not been fulfilled. If an institution is in existence to benefit the public, it has a responsibility to be open and forthright. A lawyer discharges his legal obligation by informing the hospital's management that patients must be informed of the error, either by direct communication with the patients or communication with the patient's physician. The ethical responsibility of the hospital management may not have been discharged without the hospital's direct contact with the patient. Whether the patient was actually harmed or there exists a very low percentage of harm in the future, is irrelevant.

ROLLING MEADOWS COMMUNITY HOSPITAL

The scenario at Rolling Meadows Community Hospital is filled with ambiguities. The lawyer listening to the CEO's description of his relationship with the postgraduate fellow could only wonder why the governing board would consider the CEO's actions as adverse to the institution. Although the CEO was imprudent in disclosing his personal feelings for the fellow and his assumption of what the future may hold, he addressed the situation in a timely manner.

It could be argued that an employee-employer relationship had not yet been established and the primary question remaining would be whether the CEO discriminated against the fellow since her sex placed her in a protected class. From a legal perspective, if the CEO does not hire another person to fill the position aspired to by the fellow, or declares that such a position is no longer needed by the organization, it is highly improbable a violation of any statute or common law occurred. Similarly, a claim of sexual harassment fails since there is no indication of sexual contact or the presence of a hostile work environment, and it appears any covert or overt actions of the CEO were not unwelcome by the fellow. In fact, from a legal perspective, it would be persuasive to argue before a jury that by his actions the CEO was, in fact, avoiding the possibility of a future claim.

A more disturbing aspect of the case analysis is the action of the governing board. Any decision made by the governing board adverse to the career of the CEO could be legally actionable. Although the CEO is undoubtedly an employee "at will," there are various legal theories which could be employed to maintain a legal action against the institution for discharge under these circumstances. For reference, an "at will" employee is one who is employed at the discretion of the employer and may be discharged under any circumstances for any reason.

QUAL PLUS HMO

Similarly, the governing board committee's position in Qual Plus HMO leads to legal and ethical questions concerning the authority and action of the institution itself. A clear conflict of interest exists when a member of the governing board committee participates in a decision concerning bids for construction while a financial interest of that same member is at stake. The COO had knowledge of the relationship and had a legal duty, based upon his employment with a public corporation, to request this member of the governing board committee to abstain from committee participation when actions relating to construction were considered and to inform the CEO of the conflict. In this case, he did inform the CEO who refused to discuss the action of the committee.

Legally, the COO had discharged his duties. His lawyer would advise him to document the occurrences and proceedings. However, from an ethical point of view, the CEO and the COO should be compelled to submit the issue to the ethics committee of the organization or to directly inform the governing board. As noted, the COO did attempt to present the issue to the ethics committee, informally, and was rebuffed. The COO should have formally requested the ethics committee to consider the issue forcing a decision for or against his opinion. His ethical responsibility would be discharged once that decision was made. If a formal request is rejected without an ethics committee decision, an ethical argument can be made that the COO is required to make direct communication with the governing board. Although the CEO looked unfavorably on this proposed action, the COO may not be protected from possible litigation if the information concerning the conflict of interest later becomes public knowledge. His responsibility rests with the internal description of his duties and responsibilities. Clearly, the CEO has exposed himself to the legal ramifications of allowing a fraudulent bidding process to continue and as the outer ego of the health maintenance organization, the health maintenance organization itself then becomes responsible.

A formal request by the COO to the ethics committee, in an effort to resolve the issue of conflict of interest, was and is the appropriate method of addressing the issue. This case study is a perfect example of the formal use of an ethics committee to facilitate the fair and impartial adjudication of internal ethical violations. The COO should not have retreated from his position with the rejection of his informal request. The COO was responsible for the fair and equitable application of the decisions of the governing board committee and had an ethical responsibility to expose any known conflicts of interest. Although his employment may have been in jeopardy, the appropriate course for the COO to follow should not have resulted in any adverse reaction from the governing board. The board had a legal responsibility, once informed of a possible conflict of interest, to investigate the same and promulgate decisions based on the investigation. This decision, pro or con, is the shield for the COO if, at a later time, the conflict of interest is exposed through a third party. To avoid the COO's legal and ethical dilemma, full disclosure to all levels of authority is required.

HILLSIDE COUNTY MEDICAL CENTER

Finally, the legal definition of standard of care in the performance of providing medical care, is essential to the analysis of Hillside County Medical Center. By definition, the standard of care for physicians is "that standard which a reasonable physician would adhere to when providing medical care within his specialty under similar circumstances that other specialists within that same field would adhere to nationally."

A medical institution is held to a similar standard since its liability is created through its employee physicians, agent physicians, or other auxiliary medical care personnel. Although the standard may change from a professional standard to an ordinary negligence standard, depending upon the expertise of the individual, the institution is still responsible for its employees.

Using this legal premise, a workforce reduction because of economic considerations or labor unrest is not a defense to a breach of the standard of care in delivering medical care. Legally, a reduction in workforce requires an equal reduction in the number of patients compatible with the reduction of the workforce. The legal and ethical responsibility of the medical care providers is synonymous under these conditions. Legally, the medical care providers are required to follow the standard of care, and ethically the medical care providers must follow the general principle that each patient is to be provided adequate care for a medical condition. Simply stated, too many patients with too few medical providers establishes a breach in both ethics and in the standard of care.

"Do no harm" is still a recognized premise for legal and ethical actions of medical care providers.

THE ETHICS OF MANAGING PEOPLE

INTRODUCTION

Throughout this book, the cases and the ethical dilemmas presented all have one thing in common—they all deal with the interrelationships of people and the different values, special interests, and goals that each person brings to the workplace. It should be no surprise, therefore, that there are conflicts and ethical dilemmas that arise.

The cases presented here are illustrative of the myriad of interpersonal conflicts that exist and the ethical dilemmas that may ensue within the healthcare delivery setting. Paradise Hills Medical Center is an example of the complex relationships of physicians who deliver patient care and administrators who must manage the delivery of patient care. Qual Plus HMO examines the governing board's relationship with top management and probes the question as to whether top management does, in fact, "serve at the pleasure of the board." Rolling Meadows Community Hospital looks at the "superior-subordinate" relationship and the dynamic of professional power. University Hospital looks at professional relationships and the complexities of collegial interaction. And finally, Hillside County Medical Center demonstrates the importance of the relationships between management and unionized employees, and management and the medical staff especially in times of financial crisis. All of these cases point out the need for managers at every level to employ ethical practices in their management of people.

Healthcare managers often find the management of people to be the most difficult part of their jobs. Mastering skills in finance, planning, marketing, information systems, and the like seems to be less difficult for most managers than dealing with the problems and conflicts that people introduce into the work environment. Complicating things even more is the diversity of today's workforce and the different values, ethics, and cultural perspectives with which each employee views the world. Healthcare with its preponderance of professionals and clinicians introduces yet more ambiguities into this environment. Clinicians and professionals typically bring their own codes of conduct to the workplace and most often manifest their primary loyalty to their professions and the patients and clients they serve. While this may be commendable, it does not always translate to strong ethical practices in relationship to staff or colleagues.

No wonder that healthcare managers often want to just "get the job done" without the time-consuming messiness of having to negotiate, motivate, coordinate, evaluate, delegate, educate, and communicate with people.

What does all of this have to do with ethics? Healthcare managers are usually acutely aware of their ethical responsibilities to patients, clients, the organization, and the community. For the most part, they are aware of what are considered ethical business practices. Too often, however, they may overlook their ethical responsibilities to the people they manage. While they may give "lip service" to the concepts of justice, honesty, loyalty, and fairness, they do not necessarily apply these concepts in their day-to-day management of the people who report to them. However, successful executives routinely practice ethical principles and management strategies that reflect these concepts. These executives have found that practical strategies can be incorporated into the daily management of people that reinforce and routinize ethical principles. Such strategies include, but are not limited to, management style, role modeling, and culture, recruitment and hiring practices, performance evaluation, team building, firing practices, and references.

Management Style, Role Modeling, and Culture

Healthcare managers at whatever level in the organization have control over their sphere of influence and would undoubtedly be quite surprised at how their management style and the ethical standards within their area of responsibility (no matter how large or small) impact upon the organization as a whole. How employees within a department relate to other departments often determines whether projects are completed on time and within budget. How employees relate to one another within a department and with those throughout the organization may set the tone for how employees relate to clients and customers. A departmental culture that encourages ethical behavior and civility among coworkers will contribute greatly to a corporate culture that expects the same standards. Respect among coworkers translates to respect for clients and customers. It is the responsibility of each manager to nurture such a culture within his/her sphere of influence. While top management within an organization certainly, in large part, dictates the tenor and standards of the corporate culture, it is naïve and irresponsible for a department manager to abdicate responsibility in this matter. Every executive knows that there are often "pillars of excellence" within any organization. Examined closely, these departments or programs will have a strong ethical culture and their managers will have clearly defined the expectations for the conduct of their staff and will be visible role models of these prescribed standards of conduct.

In addition to culture development, healthcare managers have certain other ethical obligations to the employees they manage. These include creating a safe work environment that fosters ethical behavior and is free from harassment and coercion especially to perform illegal or unethical acts. The work environment must also be free of discrimination of any kind with all employees treated fairly and equitably. This includes fair compensation for work done, equitable opportunity for advancement, and honest and fair performance appraisals and rewards using the same standards for all employees. Ethical healthcare managers are committed to promoting the implementation of programs that assist employees in times of need and provide confidential access for grievances and complaints. Providing confidential mechanisms for reporting such situations as employee impairment or sexual harassment and dealing with these issues through such methods as treatment/referral for impairment or disciplinary action for harassment are marks of an ethical organization managed by those who are willing to confront such issues head on.

When scarce resources threaten the fiscal viability of a healthcare organization, some healthcare executives look to reducing their workforce as the only quick fix to the bottom line. Because hospitals are particularly labor-intensive organizations, this may make financial sense. But there are ethical implications here and caution is warranted. The healthcare organization that achieves financial stability "on the backs of its employees" will most certainly not enjoy long-term success. Employee burnout and unsafe patient care are significant risks. Furthermore, in times of financial crisis, an ethical healthcare executive will certainly think twice before accepting a substantial bonus and/or salary increase in the face of massive employee layoffs. Outsourcing is yet another practice that requires careful analysis if it means that the outsourced work is done in a less costly manner as result of "cheap labor" because of minimum wage and no benefits.

Whether a healthcare executive practices participative management, continuous quality improvement, management by objective, management by "walking around," or whatever the latest trend suggests, the importance of honesty, justice, loyalty, and fair play do not change. As seasoned executives know, a manager will most often be a hybrid of styles. There almost certainly will be situations that call for participation and there will be occasions when it is prudent to be a benevolent dictator. Seasoned executives also know that managers must be adaptable because all employees do not respond alike to the same management style. While the management style may vary with employees, an ethical manager will make certain that such issues as performance expectations and appraisals, compensation, discipline, and opportunities are consistent across the board.

Micromanagement should be avoided. If performance expectations are adequately explained and necessary skills taught, employees should be expected to function satisfactorily with appropriate supervision. If the employee is unable to do this, counseling and additional training may be warranted and perhaps even a probationary period or a position change to one for which the employee is better suited. Micromanagement over an extended period of time can be detrimental to the employee and counterproductive for the manager. The employee may lose interest in improving work output and abdicate responsibility for the work product knowing that the manager will be closely reviewing all aspects of the employee's work. Over time, the micromanaged employee may become a victim of "learned helplessness" and suffer an erosion of confidence, motivation, and productivity. The manager's productivity may suffer, as well, as he/she spends time and effort in micromanagement that could be better spent on needed managerial duties.

Personnel policies, whether corporate or departmental, should be constructive, not punitive in nature and developed with the goal of improving work performance, not just as disciplinary action. Above all, a wise manager never underestimates the power of example. The ethical manager will consistently practice the standards of conduct that the manager wishes all employees to emulate.

Recruitment and Hiring Practices

Some of the most important decisions a manager will make involve employee hiring. It is individuals that drive an organization, create the culture, and determine whether the organization succeeds or fails. The task of hiring staff, therefore, is one that should be taken very seriously. Wrong choices can be costly to an organization in more than just financial terms.

Inexperienced managers sometimes look to hire staff who may be easy to control. They may be afraid to hire someone "smarter" than they are for fear of losing full authority. While experienced managers know that in order to achieve organizational goals, it is important to recruit and hire bright people for key positions who will bring needed skills and talents to the tasks at hand.

In addition to knowledge, skills, talents, and experience, smart managers will seek out prospective recruits who reflect integrity and strong character. It is much easier to "teach" knowledge and skills than it is to "teach" integrity and character. Managers often look for new employees whom they feel will be a "good fit" in the organization, who will "play well with others." Equally important is the employee who is interesting and pleasant with a positive attitude about work and about life in general. Positive employees of strong character contribute greatly to productivity, morale, and to an ethical work environment. Granted, expecting a manager to intuit or even observe these attributes on interview may not always be possible. For this reason, it is prudent that there be interview teams whenever appropriate and all candidates must be asked the same questions by all interviewers.

When interviewing potential employees, the manager has an ethical responsibility to be honest and candid about the organization, its financial status (if appropriate), salary, benefits, job security, corporate culture, expectations of the position, and the like. Employment is an implied contract, if not a written one, and there should be no surprises on the part of either party. In top management positions, the candidate may be relocating and making substantial financial commitments for him/herself and family. It is unfair and dishonest, to say the least, to withhold information from the candidate if the position may be short term.

Another area of ethical ambiguity in recruitment is the issue of salary inequities. A manager may offer a recruit a higher salary to join the organization than what is being paid an existing employee working in the same capacity. Often justified as a recruitment strategy, it is a questionable practice that raises issues of fairness, loyalty, and justice.

If qualified, existing employees should be allowed to apply for any promotion or other openings that occur within the organization. Internal candidates should be given fair and equal consideration for these opportunities. If an internal candidate is not offered the available position, an explanation should be provided to that person so that performance areas may be strengthened or developed.

Performance Evaluation

In an ethical organization, employees can expect clear and accurate job descriptions and that the desired expectations of the position will be thoroughly explained to them. In addition, they can expect that they will be provided the resources needed to satisfactorily perform the job, including knowledge and skills development. Ethical healthcare managers will further ensure a working environment that properly utilizes the skills and abilities of each employee.

Regularly scheduled, timely performance evaluations are an important part of the manager's role and responsibility to each employee. Some managers may procrastinate when it comes to this task because it makes them feel uncomfortable to discuss areas that need improvement with the employee. This is a mistake, however, for late performance evaluations, especially those that delay salary increases, will only make employees feel that management is indifferent to their needs and places little value on their contributions. It is also unfair to the employee who may be seeking guidance on how to further develop skills and improve job performance. In addition to regularly scheduled performance appraisals, the manager should provide an ongoing candid critique of job performance that helps employees grow and master skills. It is unfair to hold back what could be constructive comments and "blindside" employees with criticism at an annual performance review.

Lastly, a skilled manager is aware that employees garner pay for work (in the form of salary) and pay from work (in the form of self-esteem, respect, and a sense of contribution). The skilled manager will seek to identify what activities may provide this kind of gratification to each employee who reports to him/her and will attempt to make assignments accordingly. While each employee must have his/her fair share of less pleasant tasks, they will be tackled with more enthusiasm knowing that the gratifying assignments will come later.

Team Building

Most managers will spend considerable time talking about the importance of teamwork and many will even arrange team-building exercises or seminars for their employees, often led by high-priced consultants. While ostensibly advocating teamwork and recognizing its benefits, some managers act in ways that sabotage the very teamwork they would like to achieve within their sphere of influence. To promote teamwork, managers must model behaviors that nurture it. They must teach employees who lack the skills just how to participate in healthy debate, how to practice "civil disagreement," how to discuss controversial and not so controversial issues as a team seeking acceptable resolutions to problems. Employees should be encouraged to think independently and express ideas freely. Employees who always agree with the "boss" contribute little to the discussion. Managers must *reward* team play so that employees place a value on its effort. They must articulate the organizational goals and structure action plans and reward systems that focus on teamwork in the achievement of organizational goals.

Managers who wish to encourage teamwork must never show favoritism and must not allow employees to gossip, belittle coworkers, or make disparaging comments about their work. Some employees may believe that if they make coworkers look bad, it may make them look better. By indifference to these negative comments, managers lend their assent. To the contrary, managers must make it clear that such behaviors are unacceptable.

Providing equal access to one's time and attention for all team members is another way a manager can foster teamwork. Sometimes a well-intentioned manager will adopt the "open door" policy and find that one or more employees will take advantage of this unlimited access to the boss to the detriment of the other members of the team. Reasonable and equitable access to the boss fosters teamwork and encourages more interaction between coworkers for problem resolution.

Firing Practices

Rarely does a manager relish the idea of firing an employee. When the appropriate amount of remedial activity does not produce satisfactory job performance, it is unwise and unfair to retain the unsatisfactory employee. A manager does no one a favor by not firing an employee who is not doing his/her job. It is unfair to coworkers who may have to pick up the slack. It is unfair to clients or others who may be directly or indirectly affected by the poor performance. It is unfair to the organization that is paying a wage for unsatisfactory work. The organization may suffer in other ways as well. If a manager tolerates poor performance, that "lowers the bar" and the standards for what is acceptable in the organization. It is unfair to the manager who will find it necessary to commit enormous time and energy to "cleaning up" after a poor performer. And finally, it is unfair to the poor performing employee not to deal with the issues and to allow the employee to move on to a more satisfactory employment arrangement. The firing of an employee should be done with honesty, clear explanation, fairness, respect, and in such a way as to enable the employee to retain as much dignity and self-respect as possible. Much has been written on firing practices, severance packages, liability protection, and the like. Suffice it to say that while the "what is done" is important, it is the "how it is done" that has ethical implications. Honesty, fairness, and respect must be characteristic of the process.

References

Within the boundaries of the law and any post-employment agreements, reference information should be accurate, honest, and fair. Fear of litigation has prompted some employers to provide no more information than dates of employment and position held. To those seeking reference information, this may unjustly imply that the employee was fired, asked to resign, or was an unsatisfactory performer. Recognizing that not all employees will be a perfect match with the position they held in the organization, honest responses to inquiries need not provide elaborate detail. Some questions may be more appropriately answered by the former employee, for example, "Why did this employee decide to seek other employment?" It is wise not to answer such questions based on personal assumptions one may hold, and questions such as these should be referred to the employee.

If references are being sought regarding a current employee, managers must be equally fair and honest. If the employee is valuable to your organization you may be reluctant to give glowing reports of performance, but honesty must prevail.

When providing references, the focus is generally on the employee. The fairness issue here, however, is twofold; there is an obligation to be fair to the one doing the asking, as well as to the one being asked about. It may be easy to dismiss the obligation to those seeking the reference because they are, after all, usually strangers. Ethics applies to all situations and to all relationships.

EPILOGUE:
FOLLOW-UP ON THE CASES

WHILE THE cases presented in this book have been taken from the headlines and fictionalized, even fiction has an ending. My favorite reading as a child was "What Happened Then" stories, and the following is a fictional account of what most likely happened in the five cases presented here.

Be reminded that each of these cases is characterized with ambiguities and intertwining ethical issues so the resolutions or nonresolutions would have had an impact on several people and programs within each organization as well as within each community in which each organization resides.

A healthcare manager will be confronted with ethical dilemmas on a daily basis. Most of the time, unconsciously, the manager will make the right decision and will "do the right thing." For the most part, those involved in healthcare are decent, moral individuals who are attracted to the healthcare field because they wish to contribute something positive to society. In spite of this, errors in judgment, detrimental decisions, and unintentional mistakes are made. More often than not, mistakes are the result of the barrage of decisions that must be made by managers who are pressed for time and strained by the demands of the job. Decisions are frequently made without the benefit of the thoughtful reflection and the required consultation of others.

These cases are intended to remind healthcare managers of the untoward consequences of hasty decisions that do not consider the ethical dimensions involved.

PARADISE HILLS MEDICAL CENTER

The matter of the radiation overdosage to 22 oncology patients was referred to the medical center's ethics committee. Following deliberations, the committee recommended that the patients affected be informed of the errors and monitored closely for adverse effects. The medical staff and administration reviewed the committee's recommendations but the administration decided not to follow it. Since the ethics committee is advisory in nature, the staff held that it was under no obligation to do so. After review, the governing board concurred. Its decision was based upon the fear of litigation and subsequent "bad" publicity that was certain to follow. Subsequently, the patients involved were not informed of the errors. Four of the patients suffered adverse effects, the most serious being radiation burns.

Three months later, one of the patients learned of the errors and filed a lawsuit against the hospital for fraud for withholding the medical error from her. Since the lawsuit was for fraud and not malpractice, the hospital's malpractice insurance did not provide coverage. The case was settled out of court for $300,000. The lawsuit and settlement received broad news coverage in both television and the local newspapers. As the remaining patients involved became aware of the incident, only a few chose to file lawsuits and these settled out of court for like amounts. The hospital considered itself "lucky."

The aftermath of this experience was characterized by tension among the staff who disagreed among themselves over what should have been done in this case. The nurses in the oncology program were especially adamant in their belief that the patients should have been told immediately following the incident. In fact, there was some speculation that it may have been one of the nurses who informed the first patient of the errors. A prestigious oncology medical group practice, uncomfortable with all of the publicity and the inquiries from patients about the medical centers capabilities, began disassociating itself with Paradise Hills Medical Center and treating patients at a competing facility. Relationships between some primary care physicians and oncologists remained strained. The oncology program suffered a moderate decline in census. Some members of the governing board felt they had been misdirected by administration. A general sense of mistrust was palpable throughout the medical center and employees and hospital staff were chagrined that they had to defend the medical center to friends and family who were "shocked" at the disclosure.

QUAL PLUS HMO

Jim decided to play the game and follow the lead of his boss and the governing board. "Final" bids were requested and the contract was awarded to Acme Construction. The relationships between Jim and Brent and between Jim and the board members who had served on the facilities committee were strained. Brent began to micromanage Jim's operations. Some of Jim's responsibilities were assigned to other staff. Jim was especially offended when Brent gave oversight of the construction project to one of his coworkers. More and more, Jim was beginning to feel out of the loop. Invitations to golf declined. Jim was beginning to feel slighted at social functions, as well. Even Jim's wife mentioned that Brent and his wife seemed particularly cool lately.

Most of all, Jim was uncomfortable with himself. He was being eased out of the organization even though he had done what they wanted. Now he wished he had stood by his principles—and resigned if necessary. At least he would have had his self-respect.

ROLLING MEADOWS COMMUNITY HOSPITAL

John Waverly never fully recovered from the incident at Rolling Meadows Community Hospital. He was bitter because he believed the board had treated him unfairly. He insisted he had done nothing wrong but he believed the board to be more interested in appearances than fact. They did not ask for his resignation but John knew that he had lost credibility with them. His wife believed that she had been humiliated by his behavior and she had asked for a separation until things "blew over." His children were openly disdainful of him. The general consensus among his colleagues, even those who liked him, was that he had been unbelievably careless.

The postgraduate fellow had sought legal counsel and was told that she probably had grounds for litigation resulting from a position not offered based on gender. She decided, however not to pursue litigation. She had no difficulty finding a responsible position. Unfortunately, her experience at Rolling Meadows loomed like a shadow over her. The word was that she had threatened sexual harassment charges. Male colleagues were professional but kept their distance from her. The senior executives limited the amount of time they spent with her. She knew she had done nothing wrong, but she also believed that her experience at Rolling Meadows Community Hospital had probably hurt her career.

Some of the hospital staff congratulated themselves for knowing "something was going on" and imagined the most sordid of affairs. John's defenders were quick to label the postgraduate fellow as a seductress, noting that you can not trust anyone that young, attractive, and ambitious.

The incident was never made public but word got around. The gossip was marital infidelity. Two of the board members who had been John's early supporters suggested that John might want to start looking for another position. They were apologetic but noted that the small, family-oriented community of Rolling Meadows was not very tolerant. John was told that one of the board members even suggested that John's judgment was impaired and he could not be trusted to make appropriate decisions in the future. John was baffled at the lack of compassion and support on the part of the board.

UNIVERSITY HOSPITAL

As promised, that afternoon the newspaper reported that an unsupervised resident in training had performed emergency surgery at University Hospital. The reporter had interviewed the patient and his family who said they were completely satisfied with the care they had received at the University Hospital and had no intentions of criticizing the hospital or seeking any legal remedy.

The hospital staff were relieved as were the medical staff, the program director for the surgery residency, the resident physician, and Dr. Spalding.

Jan was reprimanded for not calling in the surgeon on second call and not reporting Dr. Spalding's impairment. She had been found lax in her responsibility for the safe care of the patient.

Dr. Truman was reprimanded for not ordering that the surgeon on second call be notified and not asking that the program director for the surgery residency be notified of the absence of an attending physician. Following disciplinary review, Dr. Spalding had his surgical privileges suspended until he provided evidence to the committee that he had sought treatment for his drinking problem.

The publicity that the hospital received about the incident did not appear to be harmful to its image. On the contrary, many thought that the patient's favorable testimonial was most likely positive public relations.

HILLSIDE MEDICAL CENTER

In analyzing the overall needs of the reduction, the CEO determined that it was imperative that the financial challenges be addressed in the manner that would ensure the long-term survivability and success of Hillside Medical Center. To accomplish this, he felt that it was imperative that a collaborative effort utilizing the input and involvement of key shareholders, such as medical staff and union leadership, be incorporated. In addition, he felt it was essential that the mission of the organization not be compromised.

Accordingly, an advisory board of the medical staff was established and identified as (MAG) or Medical Advisory Group. Its initial responsibility was assisting and identifying the most appropriate manner to deal with the financial challenges presently faced by Hillside. To accomplish this, opportunities for program and cost reductions and new opportunities for financial expansion were identified. Issues such as length of stay were recognized as key opportunities to reduce operational costs. It was agreed that these MAG meetings would be continued on a quarterly basis in the future to define and develop collaborative opportunities.

At the same time, meetings were held with key union leadership to seek their input and involvement in identifying opportunities for cost reductions. Through this collaboration, significant and valuable suggestions were incorporated into the cost reduction process and resulted not only in a more successful outcome but also in a greater understanding of all involved about the challenges faced by the organization.

This initial success may not guarantee that these financial obstacles are permanently addressed. However, it provided the opportunity for Hillside to address these concerns on a collaborative basis. This, in the long run, may be the only successful way to achieve significant cost reductions.

CONCLUSION

As one can see from the follow-up on the cases above, there are few winners when there is a breach of ethical conduct. Typically, the problems that result touch more than a few lives. For this reason and others, it is wiser to put organizational mechanisms in place that assist staff to make sound ethical decisions to begin with. In the matter of ethics, as in other matters, prevention of problems requires less time and energy, is less costly, and is certainly more rewarding.

SELECTED BIBLIOGRAPHY

Boatright, J. R. 1993. *Ethics and the Conduct of Business.* Englewood Cliffs, NJ: Prentice-Hall, Inc.

Griffith, J. R. 1996. *The Moral Challenges of Healthcare Management.* Chicago: Health Administration Press.

Hall, J. K. 1996. *Nursing Ethics and Law.* Philadelphia, PA: W. B. Saunders Company.

Henderson, V. E. 1992. *What's Ethical in Business.* New York: McGraw-Hill, Inc.

Hofmann, P. B., and W. A. Nelson. 2001. *Managing Ethically: An Executives Guide.* Chicago: Health Administration Press.

Hosmer, L. T. 1987. *The Ethics of Management.* Homewood, IL: Irvin, Inc.

Hitt, W. D. 1990. *Ethics and Leadership: Putting Theory Into Practice.* Columbus, OH: Battalle Press.

Kovner, A. R., and D. Neuhauser. 1997. *Health Services Management: A Book of Cases.* Chicago: AUPHA Press — Health Administration Press.

Neville, K. 2000. *Internal Affairs.* New York: McGraw Hill.

O'Neil, J. R. 1994. *The Paradox of Success.* New York: G. P. Putnam's Sons.

Petrocelli, W., and B. K. Repa. 1998. *Sexual Harassment on the Job.* Berkeley, Ca: Nolo Press.

Ross, A. 1992. *Cornerstones of Leadership for Healthcare Executives.* Ann Arbor, MI: Health Administration Press.

Rubin, P. N. 2000. "Civil Right and Criminal Justice: Primer on Sexual Harassment." Series: NIJ Research in Action. [Online information retrieved 9/26/2000]. http://www.ncjrs.org/txtfiles/harass.txt, Oct. 1995

Thiroux, J. P. 1986. *Ethics Theory and Practice*. New York: MacMillan Publishing Co.

Worthley, J. A. 1997. *The Ethics of the Ordinary in Healthcare*. Chicago: Health Administration Press.

Worthley, J. A. 1999. *Organizational Ethics in the Compliance Context*. Chicago: Health Administration Press.

AMERICAN COLLEGE OF HEALTHCARE EXECUTIVES
*CODE OF ETHICS**

PREFACE

The *Code of Ethics* is administered by the Ethics Committee, which is appointed by the Board of Governors upon nomination by the Chairman.

**As amended by the Council of Regents at its annual meeting on March 25, 2000.*

It is composed of at least nine Diplomates of Fellows of the College, each of whom serves a three-year term on a staggered basis, with three members retiring each year.

The Ethics Committee shall:

- Review and evaluate annually the *Code of Ethics*, and make any necessary recommendations for updating the Code.
- Review and recommend action to the Board of Governors on allegations brought forth regarding breaches of the *Code of Ethics*.
- Develop ethical policy statements to serve as guidelines of ethical conduct for healthcare executives and their professional relationships.
- Prepare an annual report of observations, accomplishments, and recommendations to the Board of Governors, and such other periodic reports as required.

The Ethics Committee invokes the *Code of Ethics* under authority of the ACHE *Bylaws*, Article II, Membership, Section 6, Resignation and Termination of Membership; Transfer to Inactive Status, subsection (b), as follows:

> Membership may be terminated or rendered inactive by action of the Board of Governors as a result of violation of the *Code of Ethics*; nonconformity with the Bylaws or Regulations Governing Admission, Advancement, Recertification, and Reappointment; conviction of a felony; or conviction of a crime of moral turpitude or a crime relating to the healthcare management profession. No such termination of membership or imposition of inactive status shall be effected without affording a reasonable opportunity for the member to consider the charges and to appear in his or her own defense before the Board of Governors or its designated hearing committee, as outlined in the "Grievance Procedure," Appendix I of the College's *Code of Ethics*.

PREAMBLE

The purpose of the *Code of Ethics* of the American College of Healthcare Executives is to serve as a guide to conduct for members. It contains standards of ethical behavior for healthcare executives in their professional relationships. These relationships include members of the healthcare executive's organization and other organizations. Also included are patients or others served, colleagues, the community and society as a whole. The *Code of Ethics* also incorporates standards of ethical behavior governing personal behavior, particularly when that conduct directly relates to the role and identity of the healthcare executive.

The fundamental objectives of the healthcare management profession are to enhance overall quality of life, dignity and well-being of every individual needing healthcare services; and to create a more equitable, accessible, effective and efficient healthcare system.

Healthcare executives have an obligation to act in ways that will merit the trust, confidence and respect of healthcare professionals and the general public. Therefore, healthcare executives should lead lives that embody an exemplary system of values and ethics.

In fulfilling their commitments and obligations to patients or others served, healthcare executives function as moral advocates. Since every management decision affects the health and well-being of both individuals and communities, healthcare executives must carefully evaluate the possible outcomes of their decisions. In organizations that deliver healthcare services, they must work to safeguard and foster the rights, interests and prerogatives of patients or others served. The role of moral advocate requires that healthcare executives speak out and take actions necessary to promote such rights, interests and prerogatives if they are threatened.

I. THE HEALTHCARE EXECUTIVE'S RESPONSIBILITIES TO THE PROFESSION OF HEALTHCARE MANAGEMENT

The healthcare executive shall:

A. Uphold the values, ethics and mission of the healthcare management profession;

B. Conduct all personal and professional activities with honesty, integrity, respect, fairness and good faith in a manner that will reflect well upon the profession;

C. Comply with all laws pertaining to healthcare management in the jurisdictions in which the healthcare executive is located, or conducts professional activities;

D. Maintain competence and proficiency in healthcare management by implementing a personal program of assessment and continuing professional education;

E. Avoid the exploitation of professional relationships for personal gain;

F. Use this *Code* to further the interests of the profession and not for selfish reasons;

G. Respect professional confidences;

H. Enhance the dignity and image of the healthcare management profession through positive public information programs; and

I. Refrain from participating in any activity that demeans the credibility and dignity of the healthcare management profession.

II. THE HEALTHCARE EXECUTIVE'S RESPONSIBILITIES TO PATIENTS OR OTHERS SERVED, TO THE ORGANIZATION AND TO EMPLOYEES

A. Responsibilities to Patients or Others Served

The healthcare executive shall, within the scope of his or her authority:

1. Work to ensure the existence of a process to evaluate the quality of care or service rendered;
2. Avoid practicing or facilitating discrimination and institute safeguards to prevent discriminatory organizational practices;
3. Work to ensure the existence of a process that will advise patients or others served of the rights, opportunities, responsibilities, and risks regarding available healthcare services;
4. Work to provide a process that ensures the autonomy and self-determination of patients or others served; and
5. Work to ensure the existence of procedures that will safeguard the confidentiality and privacy of patients or others served.

B. Responsibilities to the Organization

The healthcare executive shall, within the scope of his or her authority:

1. Provide healthcare services consistent with available resources and work to ensure the existence of a resource allocation process that considers ethical ramifications;
2. Conduct both competitive and cooperative activities in ways that improve community healthcare services;
3. Lead the organization in the use and improvement of standards of management and sound business practices;
4. Respect the customs and practices of patients or others served, consistent with the organization's philosophy; and
5. Be truthful in all forms of professional and organizational communication, and avoid disseminating information that is false, misleading, or deceptive.

C. Responsibilities to Employees

Healthcare executives have an ethical and professional obligation to employees of the organizations they manage that encompasses but are not limited to:

1. Working to create a working environment conducive for underscoring employee ethical conduct and behavior;
2. Working to ensure that individuals may freely express ethical concerns and providing mechanisms for discussing and addressing such concerns;

3. Working to ensure a working environment that is free from harassment, sexual and other; coercion of any kind, especially to perform illegal or unethical acts; and discrimination on the basis of race, creed, color, sex, ethnic origin, age, or disability;
4. Working to ensure a working environment that is conducive to proper utilization of employees' skills and abilities;
5. Paying particular attention to the employee's work environment and job safety; and
6. Working to establish appropriate grievance and appeals mechanisms.

III. CONFLICTS OF INTEREST

A conflict of interest may be only a matter of degree, but exists when the healthcare executive:

A. Acts to benefit directly or indirectly by using authority or inside information, or allows a friend, relative or associate to benefit from such authority or information.
B. Uses authority or information to make a decision to intentionally affect the organization in an adverse manner.

The healthcare executive shall:

A. Conduct all personal and professional relationships in such a way that all those affected are assured that management decisions are made in the best interests of the organization and the individuals served by it;
B. Disclose to the appropriate authority any direct or indirect financial or personal interests that pose potential or actual conflicts of interest;
C. Accept no gifts or benefits offered with the express or implied expectation of influencing a management decision; and
D. Inform the appropriate authority and other involved parties of potential or actual conflicts of interest related to appointments or elections to boards or committees inside or outside the healthcare executive's organization.

IV. THE HEALTHCARE EXECUTIVE'S RESPONSIBILITIES TO COMMUNITY AND SOCIETY

The healthcare executive shall:

A. Work to identify and meet the healthcare needs of the community;
B. Work to ensure that all people have reasonable access to healthcare services;

C. Participate in public dialogue on healthcare policy issues and advocate solutions that will improve health status and promote quality healthcare;

D. Consider the short-term and long-term impact of management decisions on both the community and on society; and

E. Provide prospective consumers with adequate and accurate information, enabling them to make enlightened judgments and decisions regarding services.

V. THE HEALTHCARE EXECUTIVE'S RESPONSIBILITY TO REPORT VIOLATIONS OF THE CODE

A member of the College who has reasonable grounds to believe that another member has violated this Code has a duty to communicate such facts to the Ethics Committee.

Appendix I

American College of Healthcare Executives Grievance Procedure

1. In order to be processed by the College, a complaint must be filed in writing to the Ethics Committee of the College within three years of the date of discovery of the alleged violation; and the Committee has the responsibility to look into incidents brought to its attention regardless of the informality of the information, provided the information can be documented or supported or may be a matter of public record. The three-year period within which a complaint must be filed shall temporarily cease to run during intervals when the accused member is in inactive status, or when the accused member resigns from the College.

2. The Committee chairman initially will determine whether the complaint falls within the purview of the Ethics Committee and whether immediate investigation is necessary. However, all letters of complaint that are filed with the Ethics Committee will appear on the agenda of the next committee meeting. The Ethics Committee shall have the final discretion to determine whether a complaint falls within the purview of the Ethics Committee.

3. If a grievance proceeding is initiated by the Ethics Committee:

   a. Specifics of the complaint will be sent to the respondent by certified mail. In such mailing, committee staff will inform the respondent that the grievance proceeding has been initiated, and that the respondent may respond directly to the Ethics Committee; the respondent also will be asked to cooperate with the Regent investigating the complaint.

b. The Ethics Committee shall refer the matter to the appropriate Regent who is deemed best able to investigate the alleged infraction. The Regent shall make inquiry into the matter, and in the process the respondent shall be given an opportunity to be heard.

c. Upon completion of the inquiry, the Regent shall present a complete report and recommended disposition of the matter in writing to the Ethics Committee. Absent unusual circumstances, the Regent is expected to complete his or her report and recommended disposition, and provide them to the Committee, within 60 days.

4. Upon the Committee's receipt of the Regent's report and recommended disposition, the Committee shall review them and make its written recommendation to the Board of Governors as to what action shall be taken and the reason or reasons therefor. A copy of the Committee's recommended decision along with the Regent's report and recommended disposition to the Board will be mailed to the respondent by certified mail. In such mailing, the respondent will be notified that within 30 days after his or her receipt of the Ethics Committee's recommended decision, the respondent may file a written appeal of the recommended decision with the Board of Governors.

5. Any written appeal submitted by the respondent must be received by the Board of Governors within 30 days after the recommended decision of the Ethics Committee is received by the respondent. The Board of Governors shall not take action on the Ethics Committee's recommended decision until the 30-day appeal period has elapsed. If no appeal to the Board of Governors is filed in a timely fashion, the Board shall review the recommended decision and determine action to be taken.

6. If an appeal to the Board of Governors is timely filed, the College Chairman shall appoint an ad hoc committee consisting of three Fellows to hear the matter. At least 30 days' notice of the formation of this committee, and of the hearing date, time and place, with an opportunity for representation, shall be mailed to the respondent. Reasonable requests for postponement shall be given consideration.

7. This ad hoc committee shall give the respondent adequate opportunity to present his or her case at the hearing, including

the opportunity to submit a written statement and other documents deemed relevant by the respondent, and to be represented if so desired. Within a reasonable period of time following the hearing, the ad hoc committee shall write a detailed report with recommendations to the Board of Governors.

8. The Board of Governors shall decide what action to take after reviewing the report of the ad hoc committee. The Board shall provide the respondent with a copy of its decision. The decision of the Board of Governors shall be final. The Board of Governors shall have the authority to accept or reject any of the findings or recommended decisions of the Regent, the Ethics Committee or the ad hoc committee, and to order whatever level of discipline it feels is justified.

9. At each level of the grievance proceeding, the Board of Governors shall have the sole discretion to notify or contact the complainant relating to the grievance proceeding; provided, however, that the complainant shall be notified as to whether the complaint was reviewed by the Ethics Committee and whether the Ethics Committee or the Board of Governors has taken final action with respect to the complaint.

10. No individual shall serve on the ad hoc committee described above, or otherwise participate in these grievance proceedings on behalf of the College, if he or she is in direct economic competition with the respondent or otherwise has a financial conflict of interest in the matter, unless such conflict is disclosed to and waived in writing by the respondent.

11. All information obtained, reviewed, discussed and otherwise used or developed in a grievance proceeding that is not otherwise publicly known, publicly available, or part of the public domain is considered to be privileged and strictly confidential information of the College, and is not to be disclosed to anyone outside of the grievance proceeding except as determined by the Board of Governors or as required by law; provided, however, that an individual's membership status is not confidential and may be made available to the public upon request.

Appendix II

Ethics Committee Action

Once the grievance proceeding has been initiated, the Ethics Committee may take any of the following actions based upon its findings:

1. Determine the grievance complaint to be invalid.

2. Dismiss the grievance complaint.
3. Recommend censure.
4. Recommend transfer to inactive status for a specified minimum period of time.
5. Recommend expulsion.

Note

Appendices I and II, entitled "American College of Healthcare Executives Grievance Procedure" and "Ethics Committee Action," respectively, are a material part of this Code of Ethics and are incorporated herein by reference.

AMERICAN HOSPITAL ASSOCIATION MANAGEMENT ADVISORY
Ethical Conduct for Health Care Institutions

Introduction

Health care institutions,* by virtue of their roles as health care providers, employers, and community health resources, have special responsibilities for ethical conduct and ethical practices that go beyond meeting minimum legal and regulatory standards. Their broad range of patient care, education, public health, social service, and business functions is essential to the health and well-being of their communities. These roles and functions demand that health care organizations conduct themselves in an ethical manner that emphasizes a basic community service orientation and justifies the public trust. The health care institution's mission and values should be embodied in all its programs, services, and activities.

Because health care organizations must frequently seek a balance among the interests and values of individuals, the institution, and society, they often face ethical dilemmas in meeting the needs of their patients and their communities. This advisory is intended to assist members of the American Hospital Association to better identify and understand the ethical aspects and implications of institution policies and practices. It is offered with the understanding that each institution's leadership in making policy and decisions must take into account the needs and values of the institution, its physicians, other caregivers, and employees and those of individual patients, their families, and the community as a whole.

The governing board of the institution is responsible for establishing and periodically evaluating the ethical standards that guide institutional policies and practices. The governing board must also assure that its own policies, practices, and members comply with both legal and ethical standards of behavior. The chief executive officer is responsible for assuring that hospital medical staff, employees, and volunteers and auxilians understand and adhere to these standards and for promoting a hospital environment sensitive to differing values and conducive to ethical behavior.

This advisory examines the hospital's ethical responsibilities to its community and patients as well as those deriving from its organizational roles as employer and business entity. Although explicit responsibilities also are included in legal and accreditation requirements, it should be remembered that legal, accreditation, and ethical obligations often overlap and that ethical obligations often extend beyond legal and accreditation requirements.

Community Role

- Health care institutions should be concerned with the overall health status of their communities while continuing to provide direct patient services. They should take a leadership role in enhancing public health and continuity of care in the community by communicating and working with other health care and social agencies to improve the availability and provision of health promotion, education, and patient care services.
- Health care institutions are responsible for fair and effective use of available health care delivery resources to promote access to comprehensive and affordable health care services of high quality. This responsibility extends beyond the resources of the given institution to include efforts to coordinate with other health care organizations and professionals and to share in community solutions for providing care for the medically indigent and others in need of specific health services.
- All health care institutions are responsible for meeting community service obligations which may include special initiatives for care for the poor and uninsured, provision of needed medical or social services, education, and various programs designed to meet the specific needs of their communities.

- Health care institutions, being dependent upon community confidence and support, are accountable to the public, and therefore their communications and disclosure of information and data related to the institution should be clear, accurate, and sufficiently complete to assure that it is not misleading. Such disclosure should be aimed primarily at better public understanding of health issues, the services available to prevent and treat illness, and patient rights and responsibilities relating to health care decisions.

- Advertising may be used to advance the health care organization's goals and objectives and should, in all cases, support the mission of the health care organization. Advertising may be used to educate the public, to report to the community, to increase awareness of available services, to increase support for the organization, and to recruit employees. Health care advertising should be truthful, fair, accurate, complete, and sensitive to the health care needs of the public. False or misleading statements, or statements that might lead the uninformed to draw false conclusions about the health care facility, its competitors, or other health care providers are unacceptable and unethical.**

- As health care institutions operate in an increasingly challenging environment, they should consider the overall welfare of their communities and their own missions in determining their activities, service mixes, and business. Health care organizations should be particularly sensitive to potential conflicts of interests involving individuals or groups associated with the medical staff, governing board, or executive management. Examples of such conflicts include ownership or other financial interests in competing provider organizations or groups contracting with the health care institution.

Patient's Care

- Health care institutions are responsible for providing each patient with care that is both appropriate and necessary for the patient's condition. Development and maintenance of organized programs for utilization review and quality improvement and of procedures to verify the credentials of physicians and other health professionals are basic to this obligation.

- Health care institutions in conjunction with attending physicians are responsible for assuring reasonable continuity of care and for informing patients of patient care alternatives when acute care is no longer needed.

- Health care institutions should ensure that the health care professionals and organizations with which they are formally or informally affiliated have appropriate credentials and/or accreditation and participate in organized programs to assess and assure continuous improvement in quality of care.
- Health care institutions should have policies and practices that assure the patient transfers are medically appropriate and legally permissible. Health care institutions should inform patients of the need for and alternatives to such transfers.
- Health care institutions should have policies and practices that support informed consent for diagnostic and therapeutic procedures and use of advance directives. Policies and practices must respect and promote the patient's responsibility for decision making.
- Health care institutions are responsible for assuring confidentiality of patient-specific information. They are responsible for providing safeguards to prevent unauthorized release of information and establishing procedures for authorizing release of data.
- Health care institutions should assure that the psychological, social, spiritual, and physical needs and cultural beliefs and practices of patients and families are respected and should promote employee and medical staff sensitivity to the full range of such needs and practices. The religious and social beliefs and customs of patients should be accommodated whenever possible.
- Health care institutions should have specific mechanisms or procedures to resolve conflicting values and ethical dilemmas as well as complaints and disputes among patients/their families, medical staff, employees, the institution, and the community.

Organizational Conduct

- The policies and practices of health care institutions should respect and support the professional ethical codes*** and responsibilities of their employees and medical staff members and be sensitive to institutional decisions that employees might interpret as compromising their ability to provide high-quality health care.
- Health care institutions should provide for fair and equitably-administered employee compensation, benefits, and other policies and practices.
- To the extent possible and consistent with the ethical commitments of the institution, health care institutions should accommodate the desires of employees and medical staff to embody religious and/or moral values in their professional activities.
- Health care institutions should have written policies on conflict of interest that apply to officers, governing board members, and

medical staff, as well as others who may make or influence decisions for or on behalf of the institution, including contract employees. Particular attention should be given to potential conflicts related to referral sources, vendors, competing health care services, and investments. These policies should recognize that individuals in decision-making or administrative positions often have duality of interests that may not always present conflicts. But they should provide mechanisms for identifying and addressing dualities when they do exist.

• Health care institutions should communicate their mission, values, and priorities to their employees and volunteers, whose patient care and service activities are the most visible embodiment of the institution's ethical commitments and values.

AHA Resources

The American Hospital Association developed its first "code of ethics" for health care institution called *Guidelines on Ethical Conduct and Relationships for Health Care Institutions* in 1973 as a complement to the code of ethics for hospital executives (available from the American College of Healthcare Executives). This management advisory is the most current version of this code. The AHA and its members are committed to regular review and updating of this advisory to assure that it is responsive to contemporary ethical issues facing health care institutions.

This advisory identifies the major areas affecting the ethical conduct of health care institutions. It would be impossible for one advisory document to detail all of the factors and issues relating to each area. Additional information and guidance is available in the following AHA management advisories:

A Patient's Bill of Rights
Advertising
Discharge Planning
Disclosure of Financial and Operating Information
Disclosure of Medical Record Information
Establishment of an Employee Grievance Procedure
Ethics Committees
Imperatives of Hospital Leadership
Physician Involvement in Governance
Quality Management
Resolution of Conflicts of Interest
The Patient's Choice of Treatment Options

Verifying Physician Credentials
Verifying Credentials of Medical Students and Residents
The following AHA publications may also be useful:
Values in Conflict: Resolving Ethical Issues in Hospital Care (AHA
#025002)
*Effective DNR Policies: Development, Revision, and
Implementation* [out of print]
Hospital Ethics newsletter [no longer published]

---

*The Term "health care institution" represents the mission, programs, and services as defined
and implemented by the institution's leadership, including the governing board, executive man-
agement, and medical staff leadership. See also management advisories on *Imperatives of Hospital
Leadership, Role and Functions of Hospital Executive Management, Role and Functions of the Hospital
Governing Board,* and *Role and Functions of the Hospital Medical Staff.*
**Adapted from the AHA Management Advisory on Advertising, 1990.
***For example, the *American College of Healthcare Executives' Code of Ethics,* and professional
codes of nursing, medicine, etc.
This advisory was received by the AHA Technical on Biomedical Ethics and approved by the
Institutional Practices Committee in 1992.

AMERICAN COLLEGE OF HEALTHCARE EXECUTIVES POLICY STATEMENTS

Impaired Healthcare Executives

February 1991
March 1995 (revised)
November 2000 (revised)

Statement of the Issue

The American College of Healthcare Executives recognizes that impairment in the form of alcoholism, substance abuse, chemical dependency, mental/emotional instability, or senility is a problem that affects all of society. Substance abuse is a pervasive problem in today's society, affecting individuals of all ages and in all walks of life. Mental/emotional instability and senility are also problems that cross all boundaries in society.

Impaired healthcare executives affect not only themselves and their families, but they also have a significant impact on their profession; their professional society; their organizations, colleagues, patients, clients, and others served; their communities; and society as a whole. Impairment typically leads to misconduct in the form of incompetence and unsafe or unprofessional behavior, which can also lead to substantial costs associated with loss of productivity and errors in judgment.

The impaired healthcare executive can damage the public image of his or her organization of employment. Public confidence in the organization diminishes if it appears that the organization is not being managed with consistently high standards of professional and ethical practice. This lack of public confidence may cause the community to deem the organization unworthy of its support.

Society expects healthcare executives to practice the standards of good health that they advocate for the public. Impaired healthcare executives diminish the credibility of the profession and its ability to manage society's healthcare when they are not appropriately managing their own personal health.

Policy Position

The preamble of the American College of Healthcare Executives *Code of Ethics* states that "healthcare executives have an obligation to act in ways that will merit the trust, confidence, and respect of healthcare professionals and the general public. To do this, healthcare executives must lead lives that embody an exemplary system of values and ethics."

The American College of Healthcare Executives believes that all healthcare executives have an ethical and a professional obligation to:

- Maintain a personal health status that is free from impairment.
- Refrain from all professional activities if impaired.
- Expeditiously seek treatment if impairment occurs.
- Urge impaired colleagues to expeditiously seek treatment and to refrain from all professional activities while impaired.
- Report the impairment to the appropriate person or persons, should the colleague refuse to seek professional assistance and should the state of impairment persist.
- Recommend or provide, within one's employing organization, avenues for reporting impairment and either access or referral to treatment or assistance programs.
- Urge the community to provide information and resources for assistance and treatment of alcoholism, substance abuse, mental/emotional instability, and senility as needed and appropriate.

Approved by the Board of Governors of the American College of Healthcare Executives on November 13, 2000.
Reprinted with permission from the American College of Healthcare Executives.

AMERICAN COLLEGE OF HEALTHCARE EXECUTIVES
POLICY STATEMENTS
Ethical Issues Related to a Reduction in Force

August 1995
November 2000 (revised)

Statement of the Issue

As the result of managed care, declining admissions, shorter lengths of stay, higher productivity, new technology, and other factors, the capacity of many healthcare organizations exceeds demand. Consequently, a large number of organizations will reduce their workforces. Additionally, mergers and consolidations will result in further reductions and reassignments of staff. Financial pressures will continue to fuel this trend. However, patient care needs should not be compromised when determining staffing requirements.

The hardship and stress of a reduction in force can be lessened by careful planning, cost management, resource management, growth focus, and proactive management of human resources. Formal policies and procedures should be developed well in advance of the need to implement them.

The decision to reduce staff necessitates consideration of the short-term and long-term impact on all employees—those leaving and those remaining. Decision makers should consider the potential ethical conflict between formally stated organizational values and their reduction actions.

Policy Position

The American College of Healthcare Executives recommends that specific steps be considered by healthcare executives when initiating a reduction in force process to support consistency between stated organizational values and those demonstrated during and after the process. Among these steps are the following:

- Provide timely, accurate, clear, and consistent information to the stakeholders when staff reductions become necessary;
- Review values expressed in mission and value statements, personnel policies, annual reports, employee orientation material, and other documents to test congruence and conformance with reduction in force actions;
- Support, through retraining and redeployment, if possible, employees whose positions have been eliminated. Also, consider outplacement assistance and appropriate severance policies; and
- Address the needs of remaining staff by demonstrating sensitivity to their potential feelings of loss, anger, and survivor guilt. Also address their anxiety about the possibility of further reductions, uncertainty regarding changes in workload and work redesign, and other similar concerns.

Healthcare organizations encounter the same set of challenging issues associated with reductions in force as do other employers. Reduction in force decisions should reflect ethical values.

Approved by the Board of Governors of the American College of Healthcare Executives on November 13, 2000.
Reprinted with permission from the American College of Healthcare Executives.

AMERICAN COLLEGE OF HEALTHCARE EXECUTIVES
POLICY STATEMENTS
Ethical Decision Making for Healthcare Executives

August 1993
February 1997 (revised)

Statement of the Issue

Many factors have contributed to the growing concern in healthcare organizations with ethical issues, including pressure to reduce costs, mergers and acquisitions, financial and other resource constraints, and advances in medical technology that complicate decision making near the end of life. Healthcare executives have a responsibility to address the growing number of complex ethical dilemmas they are facing, but they cannot and should not make such decisions alone or without a sound decision-making framework. Healthcare organizations should have vehicles, such as ethics committees, conflict-of-interest statements, written policies and procedures, and/or a staff ethicist, to assist healthcare executives with the decision-making process. With these and other appropriate organizational mechanisms, the sometimes conflicting interests of patients, families, physicians and other caregivers, payors, the organization, and the community can be appropriately weighed and balanced.

Policy Position

The American College of Healthcare Executives believes educational training in ethics is an important step in a healthcare executive's lifelong commitment to high ethical conduct, both personally and professionally. Further, the College supports the development of organizational mechanisms that enable healthcare executives to appropriately and expeditiously address ethical dilemmas. The College encourages its members as leaders in their organizations and the communities their organizations serve, to take an active role in the development and ongoing use of these organizational mechanisms. Further, it is incumbent upon healthcare executives to lead in a manner that sets an ethical tone for their organizations.

To this end, healthcare executives should:

- Communicate the organization's commitment to ethical decision making through its mission and value statements and/or organizational code of ethics.

- Develop organizational mechanisms that are flexible enough to deal with the spectrum of ethical concerns—medical, social, financial—and address them within the context of their organizations' mission and values. Whereas physicians, nurses, and other caregivers may primarily address ethical issues on a case-by-case basis, healthcare executives have a responsibility to also address those issues with broader community and societal implications. Organizational mechanisms, therefore, must facilitate ethical decision making as it relates to the spectrum of issues ranging from the allocation of scarce resources to patient-specific ethical issues.

- Promote organizational mechanisms that allow for diverse input. An organization's ethics committee, for example, might include physicians, nurses, managers, board members, social workers, attorneys, patient and/or community representatives, and the clergy. All of these groups are likely to bring unique and valuable perspectives to bear on discussions of ethical issues.

- Evaluate and continually refine organizational processes for addressing ethical issues. Beyond the creation of an ethics committee, healthcare executives should consider developing ethical standards of conduct and offering educational programming to boards, staff, physicians, and others on these standards and on the more global issues of ethical decision making in today's healthcare environment. Further, healthcare executives should promote learning opportunities, such as those provided through professional society involvement or undergraduate and graduate health administration programs, that will facilitate open discussion of ethical issues.

- Promote decision making that results in the appropriate use of power, protection of human rights, and consideration of organizational and societal issues. To this end, healthcare executives must take the lead in raising difficult issues; educating; presenting options; demonstrating personal, professional, and organizational integrity; and encouraging societal solutions to ethical dilemmas.

No one organizational mechanism or policy will be universally effective. Each organization, under the leadership of its executives, must develop its own processes and procedures for discussing and resolving such sensitive issues.

Approved by the Board of Governors of the American College of Healthcare Executives on February 28, 1997.
Reprinted with permission from the American College of Healthcare Professionals.

AMERICAN COLLEGE OF HEALTHCARE EXECUTIVES POLICY STATEMENTS
Creating an Ethical Environment for Employees

March 1992
August 1995 (revised)
November 2000 (revised)

Statement of the Issue

The number and magnitude of challenges facing healthcare organizations are unprecedented. Growing financial pressures, rising public and payor expectations, and the increasing number of consolidations have placed hospitals, health networks, managed care plans, and other healthcare organizations under greater stress—thus potentially intensifying ethical dilemmas. Now, more than ever, the healthcare organization must be managed with consistently high professional and ethical standards. This means that the executive, acting with other responsible parties, must support an environment conducive not only to providing high-quality, cost-effective healthcare, but which also encourages individual ethical development. The executive must also support and implement a systematic approach to training related to corporate compliance for all staff.

The ability of an organization to achieve its full potential will remain dependent upon the motivation and skills of its staff. Thus, the executive has an obligation to accomplish the organization's mission in a manner that respects the values of individuals and maximizes their contributions.

Policy Position

The American College of Healthcare Executives believes that all health-care executives have an ethical and professional obligation to employees of the organizations they manage to create a working environment that supports, but is not limited to:

- Responsible employee ethical conduct and behavior;
- Free expression of ethical concerns and mechanisms for discussing and addressing such concerns without retribution;
- Freedom from all harassment, coercion, and discrimination;
- Appropriate utilization of an employees skills and abilities; and
- A safe work environment.

These responsibilities can best be implemented in an environment where all employees are encouraged to develop the highest standards of ethics. This should be done with attention to other features of the *Code of Ethics*, particularly those that stress the moral character of the executive and the organization itself.

Approved by the Board of Governors of the American College of Healthcare Executives on November 13, 2000.
Reprinted with permission from the American College of Healthcare Executives.

D

AMERICAN COLLEGE OF HEALTHCARE EXECUTIVES PUBLIC POLICY STATEMENT
Preventing and Addressing Harassment in the Workplace

November 1996
November 1999 (revised)

Statement of the Issue

Healthcare executives have a professional responsibility to provide a work environment that protects staff from unwanted and inappropriate behavior. To this end, healthcare executives have a responsibility to their staffs, their organizations, and themselves to create a culture that clearly conveys zero tolerance for harassment and to implement and enforce policies prohibiting harassment. Furthermore, healthcare executives must provide the necessary resources and mechanisms to safeguard against such behavior.

Harassment in the workplace may cause profound damage to both individuals and organizations. Besides the potential legal consequences of such activity, harassment can be linked to loss of productivity, absenteeism, turnover, low morale, lack of trust, communication breakdowns, and long-term career and psychological damage.

Policy Position

The American College of Healthcare Executives believes that all health-care executives have a professional and ethical responsibility to promote a workplace that is free from harassment on the basis of sex, sexual orientation, age, race, color, religion, national origin, disability, or any other protected characteristic, and to demonstrate zero tolerance for sexual harassment. On behalf of their employing organizations, health-care executives must further realize that they are responsible for policy implementation and monitoring compliance among their managers. To this end, healthcare executives should promote multifaceted programs in their organizations to prevent harassment and employees should be encouraged to avoid or limit the harm from harassment. Sample program components include, but are not limited to, the following:

Clearly articulated policy against harassment. The policy should define "harassment" (preferably as defined by the Equal Employment Opportunity Commission), explicitly state that harassment is not tolerated in the organization, include examples of prohibited conduct, delineate methods for making and investigating complaints, and provide that appropriate corrective action will be taken. The policy should be incorporated into the employee handbook as well as discussed in new employee orientation.

Employee training on harassment and its prevention. Training should be conducted by human resources staff or other individuals who have a technical and legal understanding of the issue in addition to a demonstrated ability to stimulate discussion about this sensitive topic. Training should be conducted with the goal of raising awareness of harassment, clarifying misconceptions about what constitutes harassment, explaining managers' role in providing a harassment-free work environment, and finally, the specifics of the organization's policy prohibiting harassment.

Procedure for reporting allegations of harassment. The procedure should provide as much confidentiality as possible, for both the complaining employee and the employee accused of harassment. Employees should be protected from retaliation for filing a complaint of harassment. Further, if the procedure requires employees to make initial complaints to their supervisors, an alternate person should be designated to handle complaints when the supervisor is the alleged harasser.

Procedure for expeditiously investigating complaints of harassment.

According to EEOC guidelines, once an employee complains of harassment, employers should take "immediate and appropriate corrective action." The organization should, therefore, have a process in place for investigating complaints quickly, discreetly, and completely. Investigations should be conducted by an objective party, and the results of the investigation should be reported to both the complaining employee and the employee accused of harassment. Other staff should be informed only on a "need to know" basis.

Standards for corrective action.

Standards for corrective action are an essential part of any plan to prevent harassment. Disciplinary action should be proportionate to the severity of any harassment found; however, avoid providing specific punishments for specific actions. The policy, as it relates to corrective action, should be broad enough to give the freedom to exercise appropriate action. For example, the policy might state that harassing behavior may result in discipline, up to and including discharge.

Legal counsel should review policies and procedures related to harassment because of the potential exposure to liability.

Approved by the Board of Governors of the American College of Healthcare Executives on November 15, 1999.
Reprinted with permission from the American College of Healthcare Executives.

INDEX

adherence to organization's mission statement, ethical standards, and value statements: with conflicting moral demands, 41–42; gender discrimination and, 92–93; medical errors and, 7–9; substance abuse and, 108–9

adherence to professional codes of ethical conduct: with conflicting moral demands, 42–43; gender discrimination and, 93; medical errors and, 9–10

Age Discrimination in Employment Act, 48

alcohol abuse. *See* substance abuse

Allina Health System, 42

American College of Healthcare Executives, 1, 9, 42, 101–2: code of ethics (text of), 167–75; on conflict of interest, 35–36; on ethical conduct, 93; and the social good, 64; statement on creating an ethical environment for employees (text of), 189–90; statement on ethical decision making for health-care executives (text of), 186–88; statement on ethical issues related to a reduction in force (text of), 184–85; statement on impaired healthcare executives (text of), 182–83; statement on preventing and addressing harassment in the workplace (text of), 191–93; on substance abuse, 108

American Heart Association Committee on Ethics, 96

American Hospital Association, 12: code of ethics, 9–10; code of ethics (text of), 176–80; on conflict of interest, 37–38; on ethical conduct, 93; on the governing board, 92; hospital survey of, 130; resources listing, 180–81

American Management Association, 98

American Medical Association: code of ethics, 9; guidelines for prevention of sexual harassment, 102; on substance abuse, 108

Anderson, C. A., 80

ABOUT THE AUTHORS

Frankie Perry, R.N., M.A., FACHE (R), brings many years of health-care management experience to this practical guide for ethics case analysis. She has held hospital positions in both nursing and hospital administration. Her administrative responsibilities included patient care programs, medical staff recruitment and relations, and graduate medical education and research. As such she was administratively responsible for the activities of the Institutional Review Board and the hospital's ethics committee for which she developed the protocols in the early 1980s. In 1988, the inaugural issue of *The Journal of Clinical and Laboratory Investigation* was dedicated to her in recognition of her efforts in building a foundation of academic excellence within Hurley Medical Center.

In 1986, Perry joined the staff of the American College of Health-care Executives where she held a number of management positions including Executive Vice President. While at ACHE, she served as staff representative to the organization's ethics committee which implements the ACHE's *Code of Ethics* for its members.

Perry has also served as a healthcare management consultant at both the national and the international levels.

She is a well-published author of articles on ethics and healthcare management and was a 1984 recipient of the Edgar C. Hayhow Award for Article of the Year by the American College of Hospital Adminis-trators.

Contributing Authors

Joan McIver Gibson, Ph.D., directs the Health Sciences Ethics Program at the University of New Mexico and chairs the Medical Ethics Committee at St. Joseph Healthcare System, Albuquerque, New Mexico.

Richard H. Rubin, M.D., FACP, is an Associate Professor of Medicine at the University of New Mexico Health Sciences Center. From 1978 to 1990, Dr. Rubin worked as an internist at the Rutgers Community Health Plan, a health maintenance organization in central New Jersey, where he also served as a physician manager and a member of the physician's governing board.

Rebecca A. Dobbs, R.N., Ph.D., FACHE, has extensive experience in the evaluation of healthcare ethics committees, is an adjunct faculty member at the Uniformed Services University of Health Sciences, and presents two-day workshops for healthcare ethics committees. Dr. Dobbs is a Lieutenant Colonel in the United States Air Force Reserve and currently serves as a Medical Service Corps Officer assigned to the office of the Air Force Surgeon General at Bolling Air Force Base in Washington, DC.

She is the American College of Healthcare Executives past-Regent for New Mexico.

Clinton H. Dowd, M.D., FRCS©, FACOG, is Professor of Obstetrics-Gynecology Education, Michigan State University College of Human Medicine. In addition to serving in this capacity, Dr. Dowd was also Residency Program Director for Obstetrics-Gynecology, Hurley Medical Center/Michigan State University College of Human Medicine and Undergraduate Coordinator, Obstetrics-Gynecology, Flint, Michigan Campus of Michigan State University College of Human Medicine from 1976–1996. During this time, Dr. Dowd also directed the high-risk pregnancy program at Hurley Medical Center, Flint, Michigan.

Glenn A. Fosdick, FACHE, is the President/Chief Executive Officer of Nebraska Health System, a 687-bed facility and regional health system comprised of the former Clarkson Hospital (the first hospital in Nebraska) and the former University Hospital (the primary teaching facility for the University of Nebraska Medical Center). Prior to his appointment at Nebraska Health System, he was the CEO of the Hurley Medical Center, Flint, Michigan, which includes a 495-bed teaching hospital and regional referral center, a Physician Hospital Organization with 275 physicians and over 51,000 covered lives, a 221 bed nursing home, and a 46 primary care physician subsidiary. Fosdick joined the staff at Hurley Medical Center in 1992. Prior to that, he held administrative positions at Buffalo General Hospital, Buffalo, New York and at Genesee Memorial Hospital in Batavia, New York.

Fosdick has taught healthcare administration courses at Central Michigan University and has been a contributing author to healthcare management textbooks. He was the recipient of the 1998 American College of Healthcare Executives Regent's Award for Management Excellence for the State of Michigan.

Walter P. Griffin, Esq., is an attorney-at-law specializing in medical-legal affairs. Griffin is a frequent lecturer at the state and national levels on evidence and risk management and has authored numerous articles in medical publications on medical malpractice issues. Active in state and national professional organizations, Griffin currently serves on the Michigan Attorney Discipline Board, is a member of the Panel of Arbitrators for the American Arbitration Association, and a member for the Federal Mediator Panel for the United States District Court.

Technical assistance was provided by Kristine M. Meurer, Ph.D.